LONG-TERM CARE ADMINISTRATION:
A Managerial Perspective
Volume I

Health Systems Management
Edited by **Samuel Levey, Ph.D.,** *City University of New York,* and **Alan Sheldon, M.D.,**
Harvard School of Public Health

Volume 1:
Financial Management of Health Institutions
J.B. Silvers and C.K. Prahalad
ISBN 0-470-79173-X   1974

Volume 2:
Personnel Administration in the Health Services Industry: Theory & Practice
Norman Metzger
ISBN 0-470-59993-6   1974

Volume 3:
The National Labor Relations Act: A Guidebook for Health Care Facility Administrators
Dennis D. Pointer and Norman Metzger
ISBN 0-470-69146-8   1975

Volume 4:
Organizational Issues in Health Care Management
Alan Sheldon
ISBN 0-470-78275-7   1975

Volume 5:
Long Term Care: A Handbook for Researchers, Planners and Providers
Sylvia Sherwood, Editor
ISBN 0-470-78600-0   1975

Volume 6:
Analysis of Urban Health Problems: Case Studies from the Health Services Administration
of the City of New York
Irving Leveson and Jeffrey H. Weiss, Editors
ISBN 0-470-14983-3   1976

Volume 7:
Health Maintenance Organizations: A Guide to Planning and Development
Roger W. Birnbaum
ISBN 0-470-14984-1   1976

Volume 8:
Labor Arbitration in Health Care
Earl R. Baderschneider and Paul F. Miller, Editors
ISBN 0-470-15037-8   1976

Volume 9:
The Consumer and the Health Care System: Social and Managerial Perspectives
Harry Rosen, Jonathan M. Metsch and Samuel Levey, Editors
ISBN 0-89335-005-2   1977

Volume 10:
Long-Term Care Administration: A Managerial Perspective, I & II
Samuel Levey and N. Paul Loomba, Editors
ISBN 0-89335-004-4 (I)   1977
ISBN 0-89335-015-X (II)   1977

LONG-TERM CARE ADMINISTRATION:
A Managerial Perspective
Volume I

Edited by

Samuel Levey, Ph.D.

and

N. Paul Loomba, Ph.D.

both of the City University of New York
New York, New York

S P Books Division of
SPECTRUM PUBLICATIONS, INC.
New York

Distributed by Halsted Press
A Division of John Wiley & Sons

New York   Toronto   London   Sydney

Copyright © 1977 Spectrum Publications, Inc.

SPECTRUM PUBLICATIONS, Inc.
175-20 Wexford Terrace, Jamaica, N.Y. 11432

Library of Congress Cataloging in Publication Data

Main entry under title:

Long-term care administration.

 (Health systems management ; 10)
 Bibliography: p.
 Includes index.
 1. Long-term care of the sick--Addresses,
essays, lectures. 2. Extended care facilities
Administration--Addresses, essays, lectures.
3. Long-term care of the sick--United States--
Addresses, essays, lectures, I. Levey, Samuel.
II. Loomba, Narenda Paul, 1927-
RA973.5.L67 362.1 76-48657
ISBN 0-89335-004-4

Distributed solely by the Halsted Press Division of John Wiley & Sons, Inc.
New York, New York
ISBN 0-470-99111-9

Contents

PREFACE

The most important audiences of a book on long-term care administration include:

(1) managers of organizations who are engaged in the delivery of long-term care services

(2) college and university students enrolled in long-term care administration courses, programs in health administration, schools of public health, schools of allied health professions, and schools of nursing

(3) administrators in the health sector who are confronted with problems of interface and institutional exchange between the acute sector and long-term care

(4) individuals who are desirous of improving management of health and social services for the long-term care, and patient

The editors were convinced that the managerial problems of these audiences are so varied and their needs so wide-ranging that a specially designed book covering a spectrum of topics, rather than a text focusing upon narrow areas, was needed. Further, these topics had to be selected in such a manner that the book would provide an integrated and balanced view of managerial problems in the context of organizational and social realities. For this reason, the editors proceeded to assemble a selection of readings that would serve two purposes. First, the book would attempt to relate the input of many diverse yet allied elements of management useful for evolving optimum long-term care services. Second, the book would serve as a reference guide for the managers of voluntary and governmental institutions connected with the field of long-term care. Accordingly, we concentrated on those articles that were concerned with the principal aspects and issues of long-term care and the management of long-term care institutions.

After the initial screening of several hundred articles and experimenting with different possible configurations, the decision was made to organize the book into ten chapters. To the extent possible, we included in each chapter only the minimum amount of material that was thought to be necessary and sufficient to cover a particular topic area. This was done to keep the work within a reasonable size, because all of us have to recognize and live within the economic constraints of publishing. Despite our very conscious and careful efforts, we found that the final product was too large to assemble in one volume. Hence, we decided to publish this book in two separate but sequential parts.

The decision to publish the book in two volumes meant that several other decisions had to be made in order to accomplish one major objective. That is, the two volumes had to be designed in such a manner that they would be self-contained and independent units and yet would not violate the original purpose and integrity of the overall project. Hence, each volume has been structured into a complete unit along with its own plan of organization, author index, and subject index.

This first volume is devoted to the discussion of various aspects and issues of long-term care administration. Its organization is shown in the following exhibit:

ORGANIZATION OF THE BOOK

The need for restructuring health services in the United States into a more efficient and effective delivery system is a principal social concern of today. Since the passage of the Medicare and Medicaid legislation and the resultant impact of these programs, a considerable debate has raged as to the most desirable configuration of such a system. A multitude of Congressional proposals for national health insurance programs has emerged, especially during the past two years, and it appears quite certain that a universal health care program will be enacted within the next several years. Such legislation will hopefully embrace comprehensive provisions for long-term care and related services. It is distressing to observe, however, that virtually all of the major health insurance programs drafted to date have excluded long-term care and related services. The scope of any viable package of benefits remains a question. The single certitude is that the debates over coverage will continue, and various compromises will be negotiated regarding the primary underpinnings of any final scheme.

The evolution and characteristics of any system of social services rest upon the roots of our political system. New pressures continue to affect our social, political, and economic values; and society seems to be moving toward the recognition that upgrading the "quality of life," rather than the materialistic excesses of affluence, should be a primary national goal. The concept of health care as a right for everyone, rather than a privilege, can be regarded as effective only when there is universal access to comprehensive services of reasonable quality.

Management and organization of long-term care services in the United States are not at their optimum level, to say the least. The long-term care sector of the health services industry has traditionally commanded a marginal and isolated role in terms of both political and professional commitments, and this is apparent as one examines the quality of care provided within long-term care institutions. This situation must be reversed. There appears to be little question, however, that social and political progress have reinforced expectations for access to quality health services for all segments of the population. This, in turn, affects the utilization of services and facilities and applies both in the acute and long-term care sectors, although the parameters of the demand for services vary significantly.

It is a truism that the success of the administrator depends upon the level of resources or inputs—namely, health manpower, facilities and equipment, and biomedical knowledge. There are obvious limitations in the extent to which such resources will be made available, especially in the short run, and to how they will directly or indirectly affect the growth and efficiency of any group of service organizations.

What we are concerned with here are realistic approaches to improving the state of long-term care services and an underscoring of the need for their effective integration within the overall health system. This, in our judgment, requires two ingredients: (1) an understanding of the nature, scope, and importance of the long-term care sector, and (2) an appreciation of some of the more salient aspects of modern management as they relate to the administration of long-term care institutions. Accordingly, we present in Chapter 1 an overview of long-term care issues and problems. In Chapter 2, the evolution of modern management is described, and the foundation for subsequent chapters is developed. We are convinced that attitudes which result from social value systems exert an important impact on long-term care politics. This topic is covered in Chapter 3. One of the most important realities of today is interdependence among people and organizational units. Hence the need for a *systems* approach that considers problems from the global point of view. The concepts of systems, and systems approach, are covered in Chapter 4. Regardless of the environment, content, or organizational level of problems or functions, managers must make decisions. Thus, the final chapter in this volume is devoted to a discussion of decisions and decision models.

The second volume of this project addresses the important issues of federal and state government involvement in the licensing, inspection, and reimbursement of long-term institutions. Recognizing that *planning, evaluation,* and *control* of systems are prerequisites for *effective management,* some theoretical as well as practical aspects of these topics are presented in Chapters 7, 8, and 9. The final chapter (Chapter 10) provides a future-oriented perspective on long-term care. A complete organization of volume II will be presented in the preface to that volume.

We want to thank David Cadden, Rakesh Gupta, and Robert Rainish for helping in our literature search. We are also grateful to June Bariton and Betty Kelly for their patience in typing the manuscript. Lastly, and most importantly, we wish to thank our families for their support and encouragement.

Samuel Levey
N. Paul Loomba
New York, N.Y.

CHAPTER 1

LONG-TERM CARE

The major preoccupations of every society revolve around the interdependent areas of economic, social, political, and human problems. At the core of these difficulties are the concepts of HEALTH and HEALTH CARE. Without a comprehensive system of health care, the members of a society cannot be sufficiently productive, and they certainly cannot attain the fullest possible potential during their lives. The problems of health-care organization and delivery and the issues involved in providing adequate health services are, therefore, among the most important areas of national concern. A debate is already focused on whether the current system of health services, a major component of which is organized on the traditional "fee-for-service" basis, should not be replaced by a national health insurance program with its reliance on centralized government planning and control. Significant as this debate may be, there is, we propose, an even more important and neglected area of health care that cannot await the resolution of debates on broader issues. This is the field of long-term care.

Long-term care should be viewed as a critical component of

the health system because, in the end, most members of society will be recipients of long-term care services. It can be hypothesized that the motivation of the young is determined, to a great extent, by what they perceive as "awaiting them" when they grow old. If Americans can develop an adequate, humane, and effective system of long-term care, this will assure the working members of our society that they need *not* be unduly concerned about old age. The value system that emerges from such a conception will be "other-directed" rather than "self-oriented." Long-term care, in this context, is perhaps the most important component of health-care systems.

Long-term care is especially important in advanced societies for several reasons. First, we are witnessing a structural change in our population. The rate of population growth is decreasing, while the life span of the population is increasing. The result has been that the *percentage* of "older" persons in our population has been increasing during the recent past, and indications are that this trend will continue.* Trends toward increasing urbanization, industrialization, and increasing educational levels have combined with the increasing percentage of older persons to result in an accelerating effective demand for all forms of health services, and especially for long-term care. Hence, a greater proportion of national resources will have to be devoted to this area.

Second, a basic change in the structure of the family has taken place. No longer do "older" persons live with their sons and daughters. The post-industrial society places undue importance upon self-sufficiency of the individual. Hence the rapid proliferation of nursing homes and other long-term care institutions.

The third and perhaps the most significant reason for the importance of long-term care resides in the changing attitude of society toward the aged. It is increasingly argued that there is a moral obligation to provide decent health care to those who have devoted their productive years to society. A tangible result of this attitude was the passage of Medicare and Medicaid in 1965 which, in turn, created serious problems of management and control.

---

*In some rural counties the percentage of the elderly is as high as 23 percent. For a general discussion of the problems of the aged, see *Time* (June 2, 1975).

A primary difficulty in long-term care has been that the parameters of the field are difficult to define and technically, all segments of the population, young and old, could become consumers of long-term care. Further, long-term institutional services may be utilized on a short-term transitional basis or in lieu of a domicile. For our purposes the following definition of long-term care will be employed: *Long-term care is the provision of health-related services to individuals who, because of their physical or mental condition, require medical, nursing, or supportive health care for a prolonged period of time.* Long-term care services are usually delivered in a variety of long-term hospital and non-hospital facilities. Hospitals for long-term care include those classified by the American Hospital Association as psychiatric, tuberculosis and respiratory disease, and long-term general and other special facilities. Non-hospital institutions include skilled nursing facilities, intermediate care facilities, and related organizations which are usually defined to include those which provide predominantly custodial care.

It is obvious from the above discussion that long-term care has many dimensions; hence, the subject can be discussed with emphasis upon its varied medical, technological, psychological and social aspects. There is, however, a common thread—the thread of *management* that both ties and integrates the various aspects of long-term care. Management of long-term care facilities is thus the central theme of this work.

Management is the sum total of all those activities that must be performed in order to meet the goals and objectives of organizations and the individuals that inhabit the organizations. Long-term care institutions, by their very nature, represent special kinds of organizations and thus present some special types of management challenges. The manager of a long-term care facility must at once be a philosopher, decision-maker, legal expert, systems specialist, and also he or she must have working familiarity with the role of government in the entire field of health care. This book has, therefore, been organized into chapters that concentrate on those selected topics that encompass the specialized demands made upon managers of long-term care facilities.

The selections included in this chapter present some of the essential issues of long-term care. FORD (Selection 1) underscores the fact that the rate of violent changes occurring in society since the Industrial Revolution has increased markedly. The extended survival of old people with chronic diseases and the social alienation of young people are examples of this phenomenon. Economic and technological changes have produced new sources of deaths and disability, along with new resources for coping with them. Factors such as changes in population, technological developments, advances in medicine, and shifting social and cultural patterns exert important effects upon general health status. Ford cautions that medicine and public health are facing new tasks for which old methods are not adequate. In the area of chronic illness, a major problem is that since disability increases rapidly with age, an increase in the number of old persons means a disproportionate increase in those individuals who require care. The impact of technological change is emphasized with the side-effects of environmental contamination and decay. The author also discusses the casualties of medical progress through drug-induced diseases, accidents, and new kinds of therapy. He concludes by raising questions as to the efficacy of our systems of surveillance and detection and how new casualties can be prevented.

HARRIS (Selection 2) cites five major barriers to health care delivery for older Americans. These are (1) rising medical costs, (2) lack of sufficient coverage under Medicare, (3) fragmentation and depersonalization of health and medical services, (4) a greater number of episodes of more serious chronic illness, and (5) an absence of a health-care system that recognizes the value of all human resources. The author notes that planners must identify the problems of normal aging as well as of the elderly sick. In this context, it is important to recognize that the older person often constitutes a barrier to good health care through his own reluctance to seek advice. He cites the importance of adequate nutrition, recreation, and physical activity programs for both the well and chronically ill and the aged and recognizes the need for health education activities in order to promote them. The author indicates that the strains on the health delivery system can be improved by (1) easier access to health care, (2) more effective high-level planning, and (3) improvement in financing of programs. Commitment of added resources to the long-term care arena will require a concerted effort by all sectors of society.

ENGELMOHR (Selection 3) notes that, contrary to much that has been published about the growing role of the hospital in providing a broad spectrum of services, general hospitals have limited themselves too much. They have concentrated on short-term patients and neglected the need for extended-care facilities and home care. The author outlines some of the problems of assuming such responsibilities and the decisions that must be made by hospital management in this regard.

1

Casualties of Our Time

AMASA B. FORD, M.D.

"It is changes that are chiefly reponsible for diseases, especially the greatest changes, the violent alterations both in the seasons and in other things."

—HIPPOCRATES

Violent alterations in the human environment have occurred at an increasing rate since the beginning of the Industrial Revolution. From the late 18th century, dislocation from the land, turbulent crowding in growing cities, and the economic deprivations of factory life affected the health of the people. Old diseases like tuberculosis flared up, and new sources of death and disability developed, such as the industrial injuries which were incurred by inexperienced hands attempting to master new machinery. Great changes, visible in a man's lifetime, gave motives for new laws and institutions. Social hygiene, with tardy assistance from therapeutic medicine, brought effective measures to bear on the new health problems, while hospitals, asylums, and other institutions were established to take the place of the now obsolete welfare systems of farm and village. Economic and technological changes thus produced specific new kinds of casualties, along with new resources for coping with them.

FROM: *Science;* Vol. 167, January 16, 1970, pp. 256-263.

In the present century, the rate of change has accelerated. Many old problems have been mastered, but new ones have arisen. "Poor laws" and workhouses have gone the way of phthisis and chlorosis. Now we must ask whether general hospitals can cope with increasing drug addiction among alienated youth or how health departments can protect the public against cigarettes and overeating. But before we can restructure our health services we must assess what we know about the particular health needs of today. Because established social institutions have great inertia, change is slow and tends to lag behind need. New problems, therefore, call for special attention, since they foreshadow future needs.

The purpose of this report is to identify sources of death and major disability which are new or are of new importance in developed countries in the two decades since World War II. Using examples from Great Britain and the United States, we make some estimates of how people are being affected.

Certain casualties result from immediate causes, such as the toxic effects of a new drug or the increased use of motor vehicles. Many, possibly more, take the form of major disability resulting from conditions that have complex origins. Examples are the extended survival of old people with chronic disease and the social alienation of young people. A rough classification by cause will serve as an outline, since an understanding of how disease originates is the most reasonable basis for control and prevention. Effects on health may be produced by changes in population, by technological developments, by new factors in medicine, or by shifting social and cultural patterns. These categories, however, should not obscure the fact that specific casualties may result from multiple causes.

SIGNS OF CHANGE

Prosperity and life expectancy have reached unprecedented levels in developed countries during the past 20 years, but there are indications that we may be approaching the limit of effectiveness of current methods of disease control and prevention.

In the early 1950's infant mortality rates ceased to improve at the rate which had prevailed for many years. In the decade 1946–56, rates had decreased 46 percent in the United States and 45 percent in England and Wales. In the subsequent 10 years, they decreased only 16 and 22 percent, respectively. The estimated average length of life, which in effect is inversely related to infant mortality, has increased to 70.1 years in the United States and 68.4 years in England and Wales, but the rates of increase since 1956 have been less than a fifth of what they were in the previous 10 years. The progressive reduction of deaths in the first year of life, which has been one of the finest fruits of social and medical development for over 100 years, has been arrested.

Similar changes are taking place in other mortality rates. Until the mid-1950's the trend of the overall death rate in the United States was downward. Since then it has leveled off, while in England and Wales, as well, the general mortality rate has been almost stationary for all age groups since about 1956. Some continued improvement in death rates from major infectious diseases has been counterbalanced by substantial increases in overall mortality from such conditions as ischemic (arteriosclerotic) heart disease, malignancies, motor vehicle accidents, pneumonia, and cirrhosis of the liver.

In addition to these broad changes in mortality trends, some kinds of morbidity have been moving counter to the economic tide in these two decades of affluence. Although employment and consumers' expenditures have continued to rise, so has "sickness-absence" from work. While a greater proportion of young people attend colleges and universities every year, crime rates, drug addiction, and illegitimate births are increasing more rapidly among teenagers and young adults than in any other age group.

These trends may be temporary eddies in a stream of general progress or the first signs of rocks ahead. In either case, they warn that medicine and public health are facing new tasks for which old methods are not adequate. Let us examine some specific problems.

POPULATION CHANGES

The numbers of persons aged 65 and over in the United States increased from 10.4 million in 1946 to 18.5 million in 1966. This increase of 78 percent was twice that of the general population during the same period [Table 19 in (*1*)]. The rate of increase for those aged 75 and older was even greater: 111 percent in the same period. These trends have altered the age structure of the population. Since disability increases rapidly with age, an increase in numbers of old persons means a disproportionate increase in those who need care (Table 1).

Thus, in the United States there are 700,000 older persons in institutions, and this number has been increasing by an average of 15,000 a year for the past 20 years. There are, moreover, from two to four times as many disabled older persons living at home, and their numbers have likewise been growing more rapidly than other groups in the population.

Population migration within a country, especially when it occurs rapidly, is likely to be followed by social maladjustment with adverse effects on health. An example is the massive postwar movement of Neg-

Table 1. Measures of disability among older persons in the
United States in the 1960's *(49)*.

| Status of persons | Age | | | |
| | 65-74 | | 75+ | |
	Rate (per 1000)	Number (1000's)	Rate (per 1000)	Number (1000's)
Persons in institutions				
In nursing and personal care homes	8	90	57	355
In geriatric and chronic disease hospitals and wards	2	19	6	37
In long-stay mental hospitals	9	99	11	67
Disability among persons not in institutions				
Blind or unable to read newsprint	24	263	96	565
Deaf or unable to hear conversation	162	1808	317	1904
With one or more chronic condition and:				
Unable to work or keep house	135*	2370*		
Confined to house	47*	821*		
Need help in getting around	65*	1139*		

*Those over 75 also included in these totals.

roes from the rural south and whites from the impoverished areas of the western Apalachians into the northern cities of the United States. Over the past 20 years, between 0.5 and 2 million persons have migrated from farms every year, while the farm population has declined from 18.0 to 6.4 percent [Table 24 in *(10)*]. The nonwhite population of 19 of the 21 largest cities in the United States increased by over a third between 1950 and 1960. The resulting strain on health and welfare services is evidenced by the fact that during this decade 13 of these large cities experienced rising infant mortality rates among nonwhite residents *(2)*. In five of these cities rates increased among whites as well. By 1966 the situation had improved in some cities, but in four, the infant mortality rates among nonwhites continued to rise, while in one the rate among whites was again higher than in 1960. This drastic population movement has affected more than infant mortality. It has been a groundswell under the urban violence which has periodically swept through American cities in the past 10 years. Migrants into the cities have transferred from their rural environment educational, social, and nutritional deficiencies which have accentuated contrasts in health between the poor in the center cities and well-to-do suburbanites.

Recently enacted programs have so far not been able to reduce the casualties of this latest wave of migration into the cities of North America (*3*).

TECHNOLOGICAL CHANGE

Rapid technological change has become so familiar in developed countries over the past 20 years as to blunt our perception of what is happening. Greater ease of living tempts us to overlook costs in human health. Whereas the effects of some changes, such as environmental contamination, are complex and may take years to assess, the impact of the automobile is unmistakable. We can begin to count these casualties now.

The annual crude death rate from motor vehicle accidents in England and Wales increased from 95 per million in 1946–47 to 110 per million in 1956–57 and, even more rapidly, to 152 per million in 1966–67 [Table 8 in (*4*)]. About 40 percent of these deaths were attributed to skull fracture or head injury. Many of those who died in this way were old people, but there was also a disproportionate mortality among young men (Fig. 1). The death of a young man entails the social loss of his productive years. Still more costly is the increasing number of young people who survive head injuries to live for years with residual disability.

A rough estimate of the morbidity resulting from head injuries can be based on records of hospital discharges in England and Wales. During the 8 years for which data are available, the numbers of discharges with a diagnosis of head injury have increased at an annual rate of almost 5 percent. Of these injuries, 46 percent resulted from traffic accidents [Table 18 in (*5*)]. The estimates in Table 2 are probably high, since the relationship between "discharges" and numbers of patients is unknown. The actual figures, however, would not be likely to be less than two-thirds of those presented (50 percent readmission rate in a year). Thus, at least 1000 disabled people are being added to the population every year from this source, and the rates continue to increase.

ECOLOGICAL CASUALTIES

The casualties of motor vehicle accidents can be attributed to an immediate cause. But for several other forms of death and disability which may result indirectly from advancing technology, a cause and effect relationship is more difficult to establish. Public attention has recently been directed to the possible effects of environmental pollution on human health (*6*). Scientific evidence is beginning to clarify the dangers (*7*). Some of the most evident environmental pollutants which have been accumulating at an increased rate during the past 20 years are pesticide residues in soil and

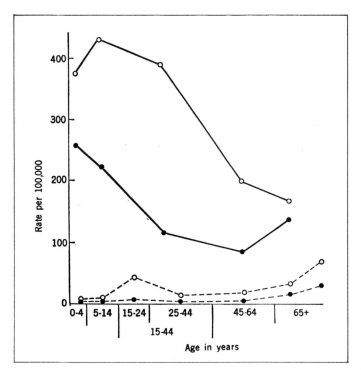

FIGURE 1. Hospital "discharges" (solid lines) due to head injury (I.C.D. codes N800, N801, N803, N804, and N850–N856) and deaths (broken lines) due to motor vehicle traffic accidents (I.C.D. codes E810–E825), by age and sex, England and Wales, 1965. (Open circles) Males, (solid circles) females. [Table 18D in (*4*) and Table 19 in (*5*).]

food chains, fallout of isotopes with long half-lives, and an increased burden of organic and mineral wastes in surface water.

Air pollution is a form of contamination which has been studied particularly intensively in the past 10 years, and its relationship to emphysema and chronic bronchitis is becoming more evident. These diseases are major causes of sickness-absence, chronic disability, and mortality in industrial countries. In the United States and the Netherlands death rates from these conditions have more than doubled since 1950 (*8,9*).

Links between chronic bronchitis and emphysema on the one hand and air pollution on the other are becoming firmer. Sudden increases in respiratory illness and death were dramatically evident in the London smog of 1952, when an excess mortality of 4000 persons was recorded in a 5-week period (*10*). Subsequent work has shown that changes in the atmospheric concentration of oxidants, carbon monoxide, sulfur dioxide, and oxides of nitrogen are significantly related to hospital admission, rates and length of stay for respiratory and circulatory conditions (*11*). Symptoms of chronic pulmonary disease have been found more frequently in areas of greater air pollution (*12*). Anatomic emphysema increases in prevalence above the age of 40 and has been shown to be more common in a sample from a heavily industrialized urban community with high air pollution than in one from a prairie-agricultural city with much lower pollution (*13*). As the epidemiologic picture of chronic pulmonary disease develops, the "cause," like that of other chronic conditions, appears to be the interaction of several environmental and host factors, including age, climate, and smoking as well as air pollution. (*14*).

Efforts to make even a rough estimate of casualties due to air pollution are beset with difficulties. Etiology is complex, nomenclature has changed, and bronchitis and emphysema are both diagnoses which are frequently linked with other diseases. Still, the fact remains that 18,763 more deaths were attributed to these two causes in the United States in 1966 than 10 years earlier—an increase of almost two and a half times, and one observed at all ages above 35 (*9*). If only one half of these increased deaths were attributed to air pollution, this would still amount to nearly 1000 additional deaths a year. Chronic bronchitis and emphysema are typical chronic diseases, in which years of increasing disability usually precede death. The price of a polluted atmosphere in terms of illness and reduced functional capacity may be greater than its cost in years lost through premature death.

In addition to air pollution, new methods of food preparation and handling, massive distribution of detergents, pesticides, and antibiotics, and increasing military and industrial use of radioactive materials all pose possible threats to human health by environmental contamination. Whether strontium-90 in the bones or chlorinated hydrocarbon residues in other tissues will eventually produce casualties cannot be predicted now, but these processes call for close surveillance. The fact that mortality from heart disease and from major malignancies of the digestive, respiratory, and urinary tracts all show positive correlations with degree of urbanization in the United States suggests that environmental pollution may contribute to other conditions besides chronic pulmonary disease (*15*).

Curiously, the casualties of technological change are exceptionally difficult to enumerate, although they arise from the practical application of science. Possibly 1000 additional deaths from chronic pulmonary disease a year—and what else? The very speed of change makes evaluation difficult. Intensive study of the pathogenesis of those conditions which show increasing prevalence is needed, as well as improved methods of monitoring contamination of the environment.

CASUALTIES OF MEDICAL PROGRESS

Doctors have always been viewed by the rest of mankind with respect tanged with suspicion, since they appear to have special access to the secrets of life and death. As medicine has become more scientific it has become more effective, but also, in some ways, more dangerous. New drugs which control or cure previously fatal disease can also injure and kill. New diagnostic methods permit the detection of hidden disease, but accidents can occur in their use. The very fact that once-doomed lives can be saved means more surviving invalids.

Since doctors are trained to be unbiased observers, they should be watching closely and reacting promptly to unintended harm resulting from new methods which they adopt. That a healthy self-correction does in fact operate in medicine has been demonstrated repeatedly in the past 20 years. An example is the story of retrolental fibroplasia. Increased blindness among premature infants, first noted in the 1930's, was found to be associated with prematurity in 1942 (16) and with oxygen therapy in 1949 (17). Oxygen was soon pinpointed as the injurious agent, and a decade of rigid oxygen restriction (1955–64) followed. As a result, the number of new cases has dropped sharply, although hundreds of persons remain blind, with only a 3.4 percent chance of regaining sight (18). More recent studies, however, suggest that the neurological sequels of prematurity increased during that decade and that they may have resulted from insufficient oxygen. The use of oxygen for premature babies will evidently have to be still more precisely regulated before we can gain its benefits without incurring new casualties (19).

The pace of introducing and distributing new drugs has become so rapid that control of harmful effects inevitably lags. In the decade 1955–64 production of vitamins more than doubled in the United States, while that of penicillin increased more than five times [Table 105 in (1)]. Ten years ago, Welch estimated that there were 17 to 20 million individuals in the United States (about 10 percent of the population) who may react to contact with antibiotics (20). Hospital surveys show that 10 to 18 percent of hospitalized patients who receive drugs develop reactions to them (21). The mechanisms by which therapeutic drugs may cause death or disability include disturbance of body defense mechanisms, cell injury, imbalance of essential materials, genetic disturbances, chemical carcinogenesis, and change in microbial ecology (22).

An informal network of clinical observations, laboratory testing, and legal requirements provides much information about the adverse effects of drugs (22, 23). Epidemiologic information, however, from which the incidence and risk of casualty can be estimated is extremely limited. The

Table 2. Head injury (International Classification of Diseases
codes N800, N801, N803, N804, and N850—N856),
discharges from hospitals in England and Wales, 1966
[Table 19 in *(5); (50)*] . Items other than total are estimates.

Item	Number	Percent of Total
Total such discharges	110,000	100
Major injury*	7,700	7.0
Died in hospital of injury	3,630	3.3
Survived with functional recovery	2,530	2.3
Survived with handicap; able to do limited work	880	0.8
Survived with handicap; unable to work	660	0.6

*Posttraumatic amnesia for more than 24 hours.

effects of two specific drugs, thalidomide and chloramphenicol, have been studied in terms of population and can serve as examples, but these only suggest the magnitude of the problem.

Absent and distorted limbs and other severe congenital anomalies can be produced by the sedative thalidomide if it is administered in the first trimester of pregnancy. This dramatic example of drug toxicity has received publicity, the drug has been withdrawn, and only a limited cohort of malformed children remain as reminders of the risks inherent in the pace of change in modern drug usage. A systematic search of the records of 23 hospitals in Hamburg revealed 139 cases of thalidomide-type of malformation in the years 1958–63. The drug was introduced in 1957 in Germany and elsewhere (*24*), and the first case of malformation occurred that year. The rate of thalidomide-type malformation rose rapidly from 0.2 per 1000 births in 1958 to 3.1 per 1000 births in the first 6 months of 1962. Thalidomide was withdrawn in November 1961. Eight months later, in the last 6 months of 1962, the birth rate of malformed infants had fallen to 0.5 per 1000, and only one such case was recorded in these hospitals in 1963 (*25*). A survey of Canadian infants in 1963 disclosed 117 cases, and 869 were known to investigators by 1965 (*25, 26*).

The toxicity of chloramphenicol has been even more thoroughly documented over the past 20 years. In spite of all that is known about it, this drug continues to be widely used, for both sound and trivial purposes. Chloramphenicol was introduced in 1948; the first warnings of its association with aplastic anemia were published in 1952; and the peak number of cases was reported in 1959. The mechanism by which this (and other drugs) produce the irreversible and fatal suppression of the bone marrow is not known, but the epidemiologic association is very strong. For example, of 771 cases of aplastic anemia reported to a registry of drug reactions in the United States (1956–66), 43.8 percent had received chloramphenicol, and 45.5 percent of these had received no other drug (27). A detailed epidemiologic study has been made in the state of California, where all fatal cases of aplastic anemia in an 18-month period (60 cases) were analyzed for exposure to the drug and considered in relation to drug sales and distribution. The risk of fatal aplastic anemia within a year of exposure to chloramphenicol is estimated to lie between 1 : 40,800 and 1 : 24,400 which is 13 times the risk for persons not exposed to this drug (28).

Thus, there is a measurable toll of chronic illness and death to be set off against the presumably larger sum of lives saved and suffering relieved by the use of one antibiotic. For other drug-induced diseases we have no comparable estimates, but the very number of such conditions which have been identified calls for greater caution in the use of drugs than many practitioners now exercise. Among the diseases resulting from the use of modern drugs are such well-recognized clinical problems as peptic ulcer and reactivation of tuberculosis after treatment with steroid drugs, persistant Parkinson's disease after treatment with chlorpromazine, and damage to the eighth (auditory) nerve from streptomycin.

DIAGNOSTIC RISKS

The adverse effects of therapeutic drugs may be a necessary price, but it is never one to be paid complacently. Casualties resulting from diagnostic procedures are still less acceptable. No method of diagnosis, including medical consultation and simple admission to a hospital, is without risk. Techniques which involve the introduction of instruments and other substances into the body are used increasingly. These include needle puncture of arteries, veins, the spinal canal, and most external and internal organs; catheterization of blood vessels, the heart, and the urinary tract; x-ray contrast visualization of organs and vessels by means of injected substances; biopsy of every tissue in the body; and local and general anesthesia given for diagnostic purposes. The major hazards of these procedures are mechanical trauma to tissues or organs, anoxia of brain or heart, embolism, spread of tumor cells, infection, drug reactions, and disabling anxiety.

Radiographic visualization of the kidneys and urinary tract by intravenously injected substances is a common and well-established diagnostic measure. This procedure has a safety record which does credit to medicine and the pharmaceutical industry. A summary in 1954 of 3.8

million such procedures reported a mortality rate of 0.008 percent (*29*). No permanent disabilities are described in recent series, although transient side reactions, such as nausea and vomiting, are reported in 5 to 25 percent (*30*).

The use of arteriography (injection of contrast material into arteries) has expanded greatly in recent years. With this technique, the dangers of anoxia and embolism are added to those of drug reaction and infection. The incidence of severe permanent disability resulting from these procedures is reported to range from 0 to 12 percent (*31, 32*). In the centers with the most experience it is probably about 0.5 percent (*33*). The total number of such procedures cannot be estimated, but active hospitals perform 400 to 500 a year. Techniques are constantly changing, and safety improves with experience (*32*).

Prior to cardiac surgery, the heart and related vessels are usually studied by introducing a catheter to measure pressures, to take blood samples, and to inject contrast materials. Experience in 16 major cardiac-catheterization laboratories in the United States over a 2-year period was summarized in 1968 (*34*). The average incidence of major complications was 3.59 percent and the mortality rate 0.44 percent, based on 55 deaths. The incidence of major residual disability (estimated from the text) was 0.16 percent. If we assume conservatively that the average number of procedures for all 513 cardiac laboratories in the United States (during 1961) is half what is reported here, there would be approximately 100,000 such procedures, with 160 new cases of permanent disability and 440 deaths from this source every year. This is a high price to pay for information, but it is important to remember that the greatest risks occur in infants with severe, sometimes life-threatening congenital heart disease. For such patients, accurate diagnosis and skillful surgery may offer the only chance.

Although the advance of science in medicine is sometimes said to have simplified the doctor's task and to have reduced the need for experience and judgment, the facts just presented indicate the opposite. Many drugs and many diagnostic procedures can be used with little fear of adverse reactions, but new dilemmas are constantly being presented to the physician. Is it better medical practice to give cautious advice to the family of a child with a heart murmur or to insist on thorough investigation, perhaps including cardiac catheterization with its attendant risk? What, apart from specific diseases like typhoid fever, are the indications for the use of chloramphenicol? How serious must the threat to life be before a drug which carries a known risk of fatal adverse reaction is used? How much must a physician know about a new drug like thalidomide before he starts to prescribe it for his patients? Surely the situation calls for more, and perhaps different, technical training, continued throughout professional life. Beyond this, the doctor needs as much as ever—perhaps more than ever—broad awareness of human values and sound personal judgment.

EXTENDED SURVIVAL

Old ethical issues have been sharpened by more effective scientific methods, but the recently increased power to extend human life raises an essentially new question which has profound social, ethical, and religious implications.

New kinds of therapy which have been developed in the past 20 years permit life to continue in spite of potentially lethal disease. Following the discovery of insulin, for example, other essential hormones have been identified and made available so that life can be sustained after total removal or destruction of the adrenal glands, the pituitary, or the thyroid. Orthopedics, neurosurgery, and cardiac surgery are now able to accomplish the complete or partial repair of certain congenital abnormalities which, untreated, are incompatible with life. New prostheses, mechanical and transplanted, are coming into use, although still in very small numbers of cases. Above all, a wide range of effective new antibiotics makes possible the control of infection which in the past terminated the lives of the disabled, the elderly, and those with chronic disease.

The question of euthanasia has in the past been largely an academic one, since there was little support among either the general public or the medical profession for assigning to doctors or anyone else the responsibility for actively terminating life. Now, however, the possibility arises with increasing frequency of permitting a patient to die by withholding treatment which could prolong life, sometimes a painful and distorted life.

An example of the dilemmas posed to physicians and society is the treatment of spina bifida cystica. This is a congenital anomaly in which the lower end of the spinal canal fails to close and a meningomyelocele, containing nerves and spinal fluid, is present. Complications include progressive hydrocephalus, sometimes producing mental retardation, and various degrees of neurological deficit in the legs and lower trunk. Largely because of infection, mortality in the first year of life was 88 percent before modern treatment was developed, and the survivors were those who had the least deformity (35). From 1955 through 1962, deaths from spina bifida and hydrocephalus in England and Wales occurred at a constant rate of about 1200 a year. After the introduction of early surgery (in the first 24 hours of life), the number of deaths fell rapidly to 815 in 1966. The introduction of this lifesaving procedure is too recent to assess ultimate effects. Table 3, however, suggests that 358 children with mental and physical handicaps are being added to the population every year, most of whom would have

**Table 3. Outcome of cases of spina bifida, England and Wales,
1963-67** *(51).*

Outcome	Number	Percent of Total
Born alive 1963-67	6000	*
Surviving in 1968 under 5 years old	2500	*
Surviving in 1968 age 5 to 10 years	1250	*
Surviving in 1968 age 10 to 15 years	200	*
Born alive in 1966	1200	100
Expected to survive to 5 years	480	40
Mentally and physically normal	132	11
Mentally normal, physical handicaps	216	18
Educationally subnormal	96	8
Profoundly retarded	48	4

*Not applied.

died as infants prior to 1963. As these disabled children advance through the school years, more places will be required for them in special schools, and many will need permanent care at public expense.

A second, less apparent by-product of improved treatment is the increased genetic burden produced when infants or children with potentially lethal heritable disorders are enabled to survive and reproduce. The clearest example is that of congenital pyloric stenosis, which can be effectively cured by a simple operation, allowing a normal life for persons who might otherwise have died in infancy. The resulting increase in numbers of such cases does not pose serious burdens of treatment or care (*36*). However, there are other more serious and common diseases, such as diabetes, in which heredity plays a definite part, and in which modern therapy makes possible a higher reproductive rate. More research is needed before we can estimate the numbers of casualties to be expected from this source (*37*).

SOCIAL AND CULTURAL CHANGE

The past 20 years have witnessed the maturing of an essentially new social order, aptly termed the affluent society. Economic productivity and automation have brought us to a point from which the total eradication of poverty can be glimpsed as a practical goal (*38*). Even now, large segments of the population of developed countries enjoy a superabundance of food and physical conveniences more lavish than those which were available to the tiny minorities of rulers and nobility in the past. Citizens of the United States have an average of over 3000 calories of food energy available daily, which is twice the minimum required to sustain life (*39*). The average energy expenditure of the American factory worker is probably less than twice the rate of resting metabolism and far below the level of effort required to gain a living by hunting or farming (*40*). Of a sample of British civil servants, 10 percent report that they do not even climb stairs in the course of a normal day (*41*).

Obesity has become a major health problem, highly associated with increased morbidity and mortality (*42*). It seems logically related to increased calorie supply and reduced energy expenditure (*43*), but information is lacking about whether the prevalence of obesity is increasing (*44*). Social and economic change have clearly produced some casualties in this way, but the numbers may be static.

Arteriosclerotic heart disease, on the other hand, has become increasingly prominent as the leading cause of death in advanced countries, with prevalence and incidence still arising. Among the several factors which define the high-risk population for this disease are obesity, high consumption of saturated fats, and physical inactivity (*45*). In the 10 years 1957–1966, the death rate in the United States for arteriosclerotic heart disease increased 10 percent, while the death rate from all causes decreased 0.7 percent. During this period, the numbers of persons whose deaths were attributed to this condition increased by an average of 17,425 each year in the United States and 3,750 in England and Wales. The causes of these casualties are not yet plain, but the epidemic is occurring specifically in the "advanced" countries and must be connected with social and possibly with psychological changes related to industrial and economic growth.

YOUNG CASUALTIES

Young people are at the vortex of modern social change. Whether they initiate change or react to it, they are paying an increasingly heavy toll. Popular opinions about previously unacceptable kinds of sexual behavior are rapidly changing (*46*), and the availability of effective methods of contraception has contributed to rapid changes in sexual relationships among young people. The ultimate psychological and social benefit of more honest attitudes toward basic human functions could well be great, but there are penalties along the way. Whether the birth of an illegitimate child can be classed as a casualty might be questioned, but the fact is that the rate of such births is rapidly rising (Tables 4 and 5). The data shown are

Table 4. "Maternities conceived outside marriage,"
England and Wales *(4)*.

Year	Annual number per 1000 unmarried females of age		
	15 to 19	20 to 24	15 to 44
1938	11.8	32.6	18.6
1952-55	15.7	42.8	25.3
1956	19.0	48.6	28.9
1960	24.0	58.0	35.5
1964	30.3	68.0	42.5
1967	35.9	67.6	46.4

incomplete, but they do demonstrate trends. To be sure, in England and Wales, two-thirds of the births to girls aged 15 to 19 are subsequently legitimated by marriage, but it is also true that two-thirds of the births to girls of this age are conceived out of wedlock. In spite of penicillin and its successors, which offer potentially effective means for eliminating bacterial venereal disease, the battle against syphilis shows doubtful gains, while a new wave of gonorrheal infections is evident in England and Wales (Table 6) and in the United States *(47)*. Young people are affected predominantly. In 1967, age-specific rates show that new cases of venereal disease increase rapidly among males from 0.03 per 100,000 below age 16 to 2.85 at ages 16 and 17, to 9.33 at 18 and 19, and to 12.58 at 20 to 24. Above age 25, the rate drops back to 5.31 per 100,000. A treated case of gonorrhea in a young man, of course, does not produce disability. But figures on reported cases of venereal disease are only the tip of the iceberg. One estimate puts the reservoir of persons needing treatment for syphilis in the United States at 1,200,000 *(47)*. Gonorrhea is notoriously difficult to detect

Table 5. "Estimated illegitimacy,"
United States *(52)*.

Year	Annual number per 1000 unmarried females of age		
	15 to 19	20 to 24	15 to 44
1940	7.4	9.5	7.1
1950	12.6	21.3	14.1
1960	15.7	40.3	21.8
1966	17.5	40.8	23.6

**Table 6. New cases of venereal disease,
England and Wales (48).**

Disease	Average annual number in 1000's for years		
	1953-57	1958-63	1963-67
Syphilis	5.3	4.2	3.8
Gonorrhea	19.9	33.1	37.9

in women; the causative organism can develop resistance to antibiotics; and the incidence of nonspecific urethritis in males, sometimes complicated by arthritis and eye involvement, is also increasing (48). Late complications of syphilis and gonorrhea do not show signs of increasing, but there is a lag of several years in their development.

Modern youth is dedicated to change, whether in the form of volunteer work in developing countries, reform of universities, or extreme shifts of fashion in personal appearance; compliance and conformity are intolerable. Not all can stand the pace. Some fall by the way and are injured or disabled. Young victims of the automobile have been referred to above. Addiction to drugs among teen-agers and young adults has been rising at startling rates in England and Wales. Reported rates of crime are also increasing, most rapidly among young people (Fig. 2). Comparable figures for the United States are difficult to produce because of variations in states' laws and because of the concentration of narcotics users in large

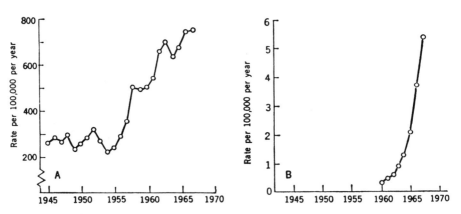

FIGURE 2. (A) Arrests for breaking and entering, England and Wales, ages 17 to 20. (B) Numbers of known addicts to "dangerous drugs," England and Wales, below age 35. Before 1960, very few and majority over 30 years of age (53).

coastal cities, but there is no doubt that juvenile crime rates and the use of addictive narcotics are increasing rapidly in this country also. From 1950 to 1960 the numbers of persons in correctional institutions in the United States increased 27 percent, compared with a population increase of 19 percent. A quarter of these—99,021 individuals in 1960—were under the age of 25, and the rate of increase in this group was higher than in any other, namely 36 percent [Table 229 in (1)]. As with increases in illegitimacy and venereal disease, it is difficult to enumerate exactly how many more young people become physically disabled and socially dependent each year because of early involvement in crime and drug addiction. The term "dropout," however, has melancholy overtones. Present methods of prevention and control are simply not working, penal systems and drug and venereal disease treatment centers are already overloaded and often out of date. Like the casualties of war, these are the most costly kind because of the years left to live and the likelihood of relapse.

CONCLUSIONS

The roll of casualties of our time is incomplete. Among those numbered in hundreds every year we have counted invalid survivors of spina bifida, patients accidentally injured during cardiac catheterization, and those disabled by reactions to such drugs as chloramphenicol. Rising casualties numbering thousands annually result from the health environment surrounding certain infants born in our cities, from the vulnerability of young people to head injuries, drug addiction, and crime, and from chronic lung disease associated with air pollution. Increasing numbers, in the tens of thousands every year, suffer or die from arteriosclerotic heart disease or are disabled by the frailties of age. Other casualties may be on the way: additional victims of environmental pollution, more infants surviving with genetic defects, more casualties of affluence, made useless by automation or retired from boring work, more artificially supported survivors, and more casualties of new drugs. Though these numbers may in a sense be outweighed by a rising standard of living, better education, less work, and less discomfort, they are surely enough to cause concern.

These casualties raise some fundamental question. Do we understand the real reasons why death rates now are scarcely falling? How well do we grasp the meaning of increased sickness-absence or the use of drugs?

In practical terms, are we prepared to cope with the immediate future? First, do we have adequate information? Are our systems of surveillance and detection flexible enough to keep up with the rate of change? Who is responsible for keeping track of what is happening and for finding out causes? Who acts on the knowledge we already have and will acquire? How can we prevent new casualties? Who needs to be educated and who will be the teachers?

Disabled and dying people need help immediately. Are we training the workers, developing the services, and setting aside the funds that are already needed to make a decent life for tens of thousands of disabled old people and thousands of invalid children and young adults? Finally, what value do these needs have in relation to our other social purposes? Some casualties have occurred while we had our eyes fixed on goals other than human welfare. Concentrated attention directed to these unfortunate fellow-beings may help to get some important priorities sorted out.

References and Notes

1. U.S. Bureau of the Census, *Statistical Abstract of the United States: 1967* (U.S. Government Printing Office, Washington, D.C., ed. 88, 1966).
2. S. Shapiro, E. R. Schlesinger, R. E. Nesbitt Jr., *Infant, Perinatal, Maternal, and Childhood Mortality in the United States* (Harvard Univ. Press, Cambridge, Mass., 1968), p. 83.
3. J. R. Hochstim, A. Athanasopoulos, J. H. Larkins, *Amer. J. Public Health* **58**, 1815 (1968); *National Advisory Commission on Civil Disorders, Report* (U.S. Government Printing Office, Washington, D.C., 1968), pp. 136–139.
4. General Register Office, The Registrar General's *Statistical Review of England and Wales, 1966* (H.M. Stationery Ofice, London, 1967).
5. Ministry of Health and General Register Office, *Report on Hospital In-patient Enquiry, 1965* (H.M. Stationery Office, London, 1963): P. H. Abelson, *Amer. J. Public Health* **58**, 2043 (1968).
6. R. Carson, *Silent Spring* (Hamilton, London, 1963): P. H. Abelson, *Amer. J. Public Health* **58**, 2043 (1968).
7. J. R. Goldsmith, *Arch. Environ. Health* **18**, 710 (1969).
8. K. Biersteker, *ibid*, p. 531; L. Breslow, *ibid.* 8, 24 (1963), p. 743.
9. A. J. Klebba, *Morality from Diseases Associated with Smoking*, PHS Publ. No. 1000, Ser. 20, No. 4 (U.S. Government Printing Office, Washington, D.C. 1966).
10. W. P. D. Logan, *Lancet* 1953-I, 336 (1953).
11. T. D. Sterling, S. V. Pollack, J. Weinkam, *Arch. Environ. Health* **18**, 485 (1969).
12. B. G. Ferris and J. L. Whittenberger, *N. Engl. J. Med.* **275**, 1413 (1966).
13. S. Ishikawa, D. M. Bowen, V. Fisher, J. P. Wyatt, *Arch. Environ. Health* **18**, 660 (1969).
14. E. J. Cassell, M. D. Lebowitz, I. M. Mountain, H. T. Lee, D. J. Thompson, D. W. Wolter, J. R. McCarroll, *ibid.*, p. 523.
15. N. E. Manos, *Comparative Mortality Among Metropolitan Areas of the United States, 1949–51*, PHS Publ. No. 562 (U.S. Government Printing Office, Washington, D.C., 1957); E. A. Duffey and R. E. Carroll, *United Staes Metropolitan Mortality 1959–61*, PHS Publ. No. 999–AP39 (U.S. Government

Printing Office, Washington, D.C., 1967).

16. T. L. Terry, *Amer. J. Opthalmol*, **25**, 203 (1942).
17. V. E. Kinsey and L. Zacharias, *J. Amer. Med. Ass.* **139**, 572 (1949).
18. E. Rogot, I. D. Goldberg, H. Goldstein, *J. Chronic Dis.* **19**, 179 (1966).
19. W. A. Silverman, *Amer. J. Public Health* **58**, 2009 (1968).
20. H. Welch, C. N. Lewis, H. I. Weinstein, B. B. Beckman, *Antibiot. Med. Clin. Ther.* **4**, 800 (1957); H. Welch, *J. Amer. Med. Ass.* **170**, 2093 (1959).
21. Anonymous, *Brit. Med. J.* **1**, 527 (1969).
22. W. Modell, *Annu. Rev. Pharmacol*, **5**, 285 (1965).
23. R. H. Moser, *Diseases of Medical Progress* (Thomas, Springfield, Ill., ed. 2, 1964).
24. F. H. Happold, *Medicine at Risk* (Queen Anne Press, London, 1967), pp. 9–10.
25. W. Lenz, *Ann. N.Y. Acad. Sci.* **123**, 228 (1965).
26. J. F. Webb, *Can. Med. Ass. J.* **89**, 987 (1963).
27. M. M. Wintrobe, *J. Roy. Coll. Physicians London* **3**, 99 (1969).
28. R. O. Wallerstein, P. K. Condit, C. K. Kasper, J. W. Brown, F. R. Morrison, *J. Amer. Med. Ass.* **208**, 2045 (1969); K. M. Smick, P. K. Condit, R. L. Proctor, V. Sutcher, *J. Chronic Dis.* **17**, 899 (1964).
29. E. P. Prendergrass, P. J. Hodes, R. L. Tondreau, C. C. Powell, E. D. Burdick, *Acta Radiol, Suppl.* **116**, 84 (1954).
30. M. P. Small, and J. F. Glenn, *J. Urol.* **99**, 223, 1968; S. H. Macht, R. H. Williams, P. S. Lawrence, *Amer. J. Roentgenol*, **98**, 79 (1966).
31. S. Kuramoto, M. Watanabe, K. Yoshimura, Y. Takamiya, Y. Ohnaka, T. Lee, K. Iwai, *Kurume Med. J.* **14**, 95 (1967); E. K. Lang, *Acta Radiol. Diag.* **5**, 296 (1966); T. Södermark and P. Mindus, *Acta Med. Scand.* **183**, 177 (1968); J. D. Mortensen, *Circulation* **35**, 1118 (1967); G. Haut and K. Amplatz, *Surgery* **63**, 594 (1968).
32. J. McGuire and W. J. Caldicott, *Austral. Radiol*, **11**, 107 (1967); W. K. Haas, W. S. Fields, R. R. North, I. I. Kricheff, N. E. Chase, R. B. Bauer, *J. Amer. Med. Ass.* **203**. 961 (1968).
34. E. Braunwald and H. J. C. Swan, *Circulation* **37**, suppl. 3 (1968).
35. Anonymous, *Lancet* **1969-II**, 34 (1969).
36. C. O. Carter, *Human Heredity* (Penguin Books, Harmondsworth, Middlesex, England, 1963).
37. K. Mather, *Human Diversity* (Oliver and Boyd, London, 1964).
38. Anonymous, *The Economist*, 10 May 1969, p. 19.
39. A. Keys, K. Brozek, A. Henschel, O. Michelsen, H. L. Taylor, *Biology of Human Starvation* (Univ. of Minnesota Press, Minneapolis, 1950).
40. A. B. Ford and H. K. Hellerstein, *Circulation* **20**, 537 (1959).
41. H. H. Marks, *Buli. N.Y. Acad. Med.* **36**, 296 (1960).
42. H.H. Marks, Bull. N.Y. Acad. Med. 36, 296 (1960).
43. J. Mayer, *Physiol. Rev.* **33**, 472 (1953).
44. National Center for Chronic Disease Control, *Obesity and Health* (U.S. Department of Health, Education, and Welfare, Washington, D.C., 1966).
45. J. N. Morris, *Uses of Epidemiology* (Livingstone, Edinburgh, 1967) pp. 172–182.

46. Anonymous, *Time*, 6 June 1969, pp. 18–19.

47. W. J. Brown, in *Preventive Medicine*, D. W. Clark and B. MacMahon, Eds. (Churchill, London, 1967), pp. 525–538.

48. Chief Medical Officer, *On the State of the Public Health, 1947–1967* (H.M. Stationery Office, London, 1948–1968).

49. G. S. Wunderlich, *Characteristics of Residents in Institutions for the Aged and Chronically Ill*, PHS Publ. No. 1000, Ser. 12, No. 2 (U.S. Government Printing Office, Washington; D.C., 1965); C. A. Taube, *Characteristics of Patients in Mental Hospitals*, PHS Publ. No. 1000, Ser. 12, No. 3 (U.S. Government Printing Office. Washington, D.C., 1965); A. L. Jackson, *Prevalence of Selected Impairments*, PHS Publ. No. 1000, Ser. 10, No. 48 (U.S. Government Printing Office, Washington, D.C., 1968); C. S. Wilder, *Limitation of Activity and Mobility Due to Chronic Conditions*, PHS Publ. No. 1000, Ser. 10, No. 45 (U.S. Government Printing Office, Washington, D.C., 1968).

50. W. Lewin, *Brit. Med. J.* 1, 465 (1968); P. S. London, *Ann. Roy. Coll. Surg. Engl.* 41, 460 (1967).

51. J. Lorber, *Medical Officer* 119, 213 (1968).

52. U.S. Department of Health, Education and Welfare, Public Health Service, *Vital Statistics of the United States, 1940–1966* (U.S. Government Printing Office, Washington, D.C.).

53. Home Office, *Annual Criminal Statistics* (H.M. Stationery Office, London, 1945–67); reports by H.M. Government of the U.K. to the United Nations.

54. I thank Professor J. N. Morris, Professor of Public Health at the London School of Hygiene and Tropical Medicine, for guidance and assistance. The report was written in his department during my sabbatical leave, with financial support from the United States Public Health Service and the Milbank Memorial Fund.

2

Breaking the Barriers to Better Health-Care Delivery for the Aged

RAYMOND HARRIS, M.D.

MEDICAL ASPECTS

Five major medical barriers to health care delivery for older Americans documented in Hearings before the Subcommittee on Health of the Elderly of the Special Committee on Aging, United States Senate, (March 5 & 6, 1973) include:

(1) *Rising medical costs which have outpriced all but the most affluent elderly.* In my experience as a physician and medical school professor, costs of health and medical care delivery to older people have been needlessly increased by inept bureaucratic interpretations of Medicare and Medicaid regulations.

(2) *Lack of coverage under Medicare which denies needed services for millions of older people ineligible for Medicaid but too poor to pay for such services out of their own pockets.* Again, in my experience, Medicare, as presently constituted, does not cover enough critical, medically related services required by older people—drugs, dentistry, podiatry, medical appliances, mental health care, and home health services. This lack of coverage often requires expensive and unsatisfactory alternatives by city, state, and federal governments to meet the needs for such services.

FROM: *The Gerontologist*, Vol. 15, Part 1., February 1975, pp. 52-56.

(3) *Fragmentation and depersonalization of health and medical services* which prevent an older person from receiving required broad and comprehensive medical care.

(4) *Greater number of more serious, multiple health and medical problems, usually chronic, which require considerable recurrent medical care.* Older persons 65 and over visit their doctors on the average of 7.2 times per year compared with 5 visits yearly by people 45-64 years of age. Furthermore, the rate of the elderly hospitalized exceeds that for the total population. At ages 45-65, about 1 person in 7 is hospitalized each year—at ages 75 and over, about 1 person in 4.

In addition, older people tend to stay longer in hospitals. In 1970 the patient over 65 years of age stayed almost twice as long as the younger patient; the older person averaged 12.7 days per stay compared to 7 or fewer days for those under 65 years of age. Such longer hospital stays may arise because older people have no one at home to care for them, and good nursing homes, health home aides, and homemakers may be in short supply in the community. Thus, in effect, the lack of available home or nursing home care in the community, rather than the illness or availability of Medicare to cover hospital bills, contributes to the seemingly excessive hospital stays of some older patients.

(5) *Lack of a good health care system which recognizes the deeper human resources in life.* Any health care system for the elderly person must be concerned with the medical, health, psychological, socioeconomic, institutional, and other problems, including his growing alienation from society and fellow man, that complicate the life of an aging person in our society. Only by understanding what we are doing to the older person can we hope to improve the health care delivery service.

These five major barriers to health care delivery have been briefly commented upon. It is now time to see what must be done to break these barriers focusing upon: (1) the needs of the client (patient), (2) The needs of the health-care delivery system.

NEEDS OF THE CLIENT (PATIENT)

The average recipient of health care delivery services is a person 65 years and over with many basic human needs, including good physical health, social acceptance, a satisfying occupation, recreation, freedom of choice, and a mutual exchange of human affection. Any effective health care delivery system must satisfy these basic needs as well as the emotional needs of aging people, such as personal hopes, aspirations and expectations, self-esteem, self-respect, and independence. Otherwise, societal, physical, mental and medical restraints and limitations or diseases opposing these important physiologic and psychologic needs of aging people may lead to unsuccessful adaptive aging patterns which eventually provoke mental illness.

Over-all planning for better health and medical care delivery systems must identify problems of the well aged and the sick arising from the normal aging process. Changes in sensory perception as a result of this aging process limit their ability to hear, see, taste, smell, adapt to light, and perceive color and may initiate reverberations in the psychologic sphere, induce personality changes, and complicate interpersonal relations. The aging process may also cause physical problems affecting motivation, vigor, and mobility as a result of neuromuscular changes, muscular weakness, incoordination, adaptive shortening of muscles, immobility of joints, muscle spasms, or spasticity. Bad hearing, poor eyesight, loss of balance or equilibrium, inability to climb stairs, or dizziness, even in the absence of disease, may further aggravate such problems. Organic disease, superimposed upon the changes of the normal aging process, may further limit the elderly person's activity. The leading organic causes of such limitation of activity in order of importance in people 65 years and older (National Center for Health Statistics, 1971, Table 8, July, 1965 June, 1967) are as follows:

Heart conditions—21.9%
Arthritis and rheumatism—20.2%
Visual impairments—9.1%
Hypertension without heart involvement—7.0%
Mental and nervous conditions—5.8%
Impairment of lower extremities and hips—5.4%

Such planning must also provide high quality health and medical care delivery programs which not only supplies proper treatment, appropriate illness support, and sensible preventive health measures but also allows for individual idiosyncrasies of ailing people, particularly older ones. Into the system must be built comprehensive care programs which include the psychosocial and emotional needs of human beings and the practical aspects of community organizational patterns.

The older person himself at times constitutes a barrier to good health care and delivery. For example, it has been noted that many older people are reluctant to seek medical advice, even in Great Britain where under the National Health Services that cost is born by the government rather than the individual. One study of the British health system estimates that only 1 person in 4 with symptoms seeks medical advice.

Denial of illness, one of the most common defense mechanisms of ailing people, constitutes another barrier. A patient who denies his illness is not only trying to conceal his excessive anxiety from the physician, but also from himself. Such a patient may simply ignore somatic complaints, attempt to minimize their importance, or attribute them to a variety of innocuous causes. He is clearly unprepared to cooperate with therapeutic plans or to take his prescribed medication consistently or for any great length of time. He tends to ignore most medical advice.

Proper management of this condition requires breaking through the patient's defenses to learn what illness really means to him and why the idea of illness arouses such undue anxiety in him. Is his excessive anxiety based on deeply repressed apprehensions concerning his specific illness? Does he equate being ill with dependency upon others or consider illness a threat to his self-image? He may think he is not being told the whole truth about his condition. Through skilled questioning, even in a session as brief as 10 min., the physician can often elicit the answers if he allows the patient to do most of the talking to bring repressed anxieties to the surface. Counseling and reassurance can relieve most such anxieties, but when anxiety appears unduly severe and persistent, additional antianxiety support with drugs may occasionally be required. The system must allow time and flexibility for such treatments.

Periodic and screening health examinations should be available for proper health maintenance and prevention of illness. Much serious disability and illness can be prevented if diseases are detected early. Common screening tests are widely available for the major chronic illnesses of old age, diabetes, glaucoma, heart disease, tuberculosis, and cancer. Annual general health evaluations should include routine blood tests, electrocardiogram, chest x-ray, and urine analysis as a minimum. Screening programs should include an effective follow-up and referral service to insure that proper medical care is given when needed. Health programs should also include immunization against influenza and other diseases.

For good health, the well aged and the chronically ill aged also require adequate nutrition, recreation, and regular physical activity programs to maintain their well-being, muscular strength and tone, proper joint movements, good circulation, and digestion. Regular physical activity provides an emotional outlet for the worries of daily life, enhances the feeling of well-being, reduces free-flowing tension, inhibits aggression and hostility, provides kinesthetic stimulation and emotional satisfaction.

Greater health education of the elderly and their families is also an important need. Better educational materials and audio-visual programs on health must be made available to assist older people and their families to recognize early symptoms of disease. Very often the elderly do not utilize proper health services because they attribute their complaints to growing old rather than to disease or remediable disorders. Health education programs should provide details of all benefits to which elderly patients are entitled. For example, legally blind people may be entitled to reduction of various taxes and access to programs, talking books, and other measures which help them to live better, but not enough of them are aware of such available benefits.

NEEDS OF THE HEALTH CARE DELIVERY SYSTEM

The problems of an already overextended and inadequate health care delivery system have been compounded by demographic population changes resulting from the increased life expectancy of people. Today, every tenth person is 65 or over and there is a total of almost 20 million men and women age 65 or more. This segment of the population over 65 will reach 25 million by 1980 and 28.2 million by the year 2000 (Harris, 1970).

The strains on this system can be improved by (1) easier access to health care, (2) more effective high-level planning, and (3) improvement in financing of programs.

(1) Easier access to health care requires community health services of the *right kind*, in the *right place*, at the *right time*. These include trained physicians available and willing to care for older people, community-related ambulatory care centers affiliated with medical schools, well managed hospitals and other health-related facilities such as the nursing homes, convalescent homes, day care centers, visiting nurses, and home health aides. Vocational and social rehabilitation services as well as adequate housing, home safety, good sanitation programs, home visiting programs, and multipurpose senior citizens centers should also be provided so that older people can live active lives in spite of age and disease.

Since the health care system does not begin operating until the patient takes the initiative by visiting a physician or clinic, usually too late in the progress of disease, an interventionist approach must be inaugurated so that physicians and other health workers can reach out to elderly people who, for genetic reasons, occupation, or way of life, have a special predisposition to disease. Such intervention in the early stages of disease will be most effective in preventing the progress of disease.

Nurse-practitioners, improved screening facilities, and health fairs to unearth illness will also facilitate access to health care services. Better training of health professionals and primary care physicians as well as modernization of existing facilities and the development of innovative methods for providing medical manpower in rural districts, the inner city, and other areas will also improve access of individuals to the health system.

(2) High-level planning for better education of physicians and other health professionals is essential to reduce the chaotic spasms of the present health care delivery system which is oriented primarily toward the treatment of acute phase of illness and does not offer a complete spectrum of health care with sufficient alternatives to acute care; proper financing for

the alternatives, and education of physicians and patients in accepting these alternatives. Current medical care is far too concerned with organic pathology and problems of disease and too little with the hopes, aspirations, and life styles of aging individuals. As a result, many older people are expensively overtreated and overdiagnosed.

Good medical care for the elderly requires an interested and responsive medical profession, including a cadre of physicians, geriatric consultants, and clinical gerontologists versed in the diseases of aging, the age-related changes that occur in the absence of disease, and the use of allied health professionals and community resources. Such specialists are necessary to identify gaps in knowledge about aging, to gather the clinical and research information concerning time-related changes of disease in normal aging, to promote and prescribe preventive therapeutic measures to keep old people healthy, and improve their health when disease intervenes. Such geriatric specialists are essential to develop the wellness concept in old age.

One major reason for our present Alice in Geriatric Wonderland state of affairs is that too few American medical schools offer geriatric training. The excuse is ostensibly lack of money, but vested professional interests protecting the status quo of existing well-established departments in medical schools is the more likely reason. Improvement of the quality and quantity of health care services requires more geriatric specialists and primary care physicians and health professionals to care for the aged. Departments of geriatrics and gerontology must be established in medical schools so that medical students, interns, and residents, as well as other health workers, may be trained properly. Effective training of people to care for the aged cannot take place without interested and active medical school involvement.

Toward this end, high level national planning among government officials, medical school educators, voluntary health leaders, practicing physicians, and others is essential to establish and finance departments of geriatrics and gerontology in medical schools, to improve the climate in training for the care of the elderly, to coordinate services and facilities for the aged—well and sick—and to lower costs by eliminating duplication and over-utilization.

Quality medical service also requires empathetic conversation and interpersonal interaction among the patient, physician, and other specialized professionals and technicians delivering medical care to the aged. Today, the more traditional health system of a close, long-term relationship with a family doctor which existed in the past is now unfortunately being replaced in this age of specialty by less satisfactory short-term encounters with specialists and other professionals. One major cause is existing hospital and medical school administrative policies which escalate costs and lower the quality of medical care. One such detrimental policy promulgated by too many medical schools and hospital centers is limitation of staff privileges to full-time faculty and physicians already on their staffs. Such institutions accept new private practitioners grudgingly, if at all. As a result, primary physicians caring for the elderly in the community must turn them over to hospital-based physicians for care when they need hospitalization. Elderly patients going to emergency rooms for acute care are frequently not referred back to their own doctor if hospitalized; and, if treated and sent home, the results of their tests are not readily available to the physician in the community. In hospital institutions with closed staffs, a patient may be admitted through the emergency room and treated by the resident or house staff or an unknown attending doctor unacquainted with the patient, who must repeat tests perhaps already performed by the patient's own physician. Repetition of these tests in elderly-patients, who often have four to five chronic disorders, skyrockets the medical expenses. Upon discharge, the patient may return to his family doctor, who then faces the problem of obtaining information from the hospital record department where records may remain imcomplete for several months. Open medical and surgical hospital staffs are preferable so that qualified physicians in the community may admit their patients to good hospitals, share in the educational programs, and participate in the health and medical care of their hospitalized patients. Even the British health system, which originally propagated this sharp schism between community practitioners and hospital staff, has "seen the light" and taken steps to re-integrate community practitioners into the hospital system.

(3) Improvement in financing health care programs requires the upgrading of current financing of health coverage and services. Although Medicare has increased utilization of health services by older people, it does not pay for preventive or health maintenance services, and, in many instances, services for which Medicare and Medicaid will pay are not available in the community.

Wiser financing of home health services and alternatives to institutional care such as meals-on-wheels, transportation, adult day care centers, home health aides and homemaker programs within the health care delivery system is essential to help older people remain at home (Home Health Services in the United States, 1973).

Other useful services that assist the elderly to stay out of institutions could include: (1) household handymen to clean house and perform repairs and seasonal tasks, such as changing screens, moving furniture, cleaning porches or yards, (2) geriatric aides to supply companionship, light housekeeping, and limited bedside care, (3) home aides to provide escort services, run errands, and shop for the infirm elderly, (4) outreach aides to locate older people in the community, visiting them, ascertaining their needs, and making appropriate referrals to agencies and follow-up care.

Innovative programs like the pilot projects for the blind in this country have been started by some associations for the blind but they are so new that many people concerned with these problems know too little about them.

Improvement of universal access to comprehensive services requires reform of the regulations concerning the delivery of services, a viable manpower policy, proper instruments to carry it out, a workable financing mechanism that permits every American to secure comprehensive health services free from catastrophic financial barriers, and providers to deliver such services efficiently and economically.

The establishment of the National Institute of Aging should favorably influence the quantity and quality of health and medical care service delivery to the elderly by providing more monies for medical research on the aging process, the diseases of old age, and the delivery of health care services. In this age of specialty this Institution will upgrade the speciality of age.

CONCLUSION

The socioeconomic impact of increased numbers of older people and the greater incidence of disease in them have seriously strained the medical profession, the allied health professions, and a health care delivery system that is designed more for acute rather than for chronic disease. However, neither the medical profession nor any single segment of society can really be held responsible for this sorry state of affairs. Medical historians recognize that the characteristic attitudes of the medical profession are determined mainly by the attitude of society toward health and disease, and that medical practices and care in different periods of history differ according to the structure and wishes of society at the time (Sigerist, 1960). The real culprit is the inevitable lagging of major social policies behind the rapid advances in the science and art of medicine which have prolonged life.

Therefore, changes in social policies must be introduced if barriers to better health care delivery for the aged are to be broken. Fortunately, appropriate social policies do correct most of the problems (Sigerist, 1960). As Post, a British psychiatrist, wrote (1965)

> Adequate care of elderly persons in distress, from whatever cause, is a matter of public conscience. Medical workers should most certainly draw the attention of their community to these problems but should be careful not to overstate their case.

Planners and decision-makers of society, including the medical profession, must enter into a crucial dialogue on the major problems of health care service delivery and call upon their counterparts in religion, philosphy, politics, economics, and other social sciences to upgrade their social thinking on these subjects and to answer some important basic questions such as the following: How far should one go to maintain life in the face of incurable disease? How much of the gross national product should go into health care? Since poverty and poor health are so closely linked, is it better to seek improved health care by attacking poverty rather than by deploying medical resources? Such answers require not only medical concern but also formulation of social policies and their expression through the political system. Now is the time for such concerted action by all to break the barriers to better health care delivery for the aged!

References

Hearings before the Subcommittee on Health of the Elderly of the Special Committee on Aging of the United States Senate. **Barriers to health care for older Americans.** Part I, Mar. 5, 1973, #5270-01927; Part II, Mar. 6, 1973, #5270-01954. USGP, Washington, 1973.

Harris, R. **The Management of geriatric cardiovascular disease.** Lippincott, Philadelphia, 1970.

Home Health Services in the United States: A working paper on current status prepared by the Special Committee on Aging, United States Senate, July, 1973. USGPO, Washington, #5270-01874.

National Center for Health Statistics, HEW. **Health in the later years of life.** USGPO, Washington, 1971, #1722-0178.

Post, F. **The clinical psychiatry of late life.** Pergamon Press, Oxford, 1965.

Sigerist, H. E. The physician's profession through the ages. In Marti-Ibanez (Ed.) **Henry E. Sigerist on the history of medicine.** MD Publications, New York, 1960.

General Hospitals and the Long-Term Care Gap

JACK H. ENGELMOHR

In 1966 the National Commission on Community Health Services characterized the lack of sufficient places to meet the long-term illness requirements of the increasing number of older persons in our society as "the widest gap in health-care facilities in most parts of the United States."[1] The top priority for long-term patients as set forth in that report was "the construction of extended care facilities under voluntary nonprofit auspices physically or functionally related to a general hospital."[2]

By 1970 the number of nursing homes and nursing home beds had increased dramatically. Stimulated by the prospect of obtaining public funds through Medicare and Medicaid, there was much activity within this unique industry. Nursing homes grew in size as well as in numbers. Between 1960 and 1970 the number of beds and patients more than tripled, to 1.1 million and 900,000, respectively. During the same ten years expenditures for care increased from $.5 billion to $2.8 billion and by 1974 had reached $7.5 billion, an increase of 1,400 percent.[3]

Despite the recommendations of the National Commission and the view of many that hospitals should become more directly involved in long-term care, this has not happened. Although our community general hospitals are the best-equipped institutions to organize and operate long-term care units, skilled nursing and intermediate-care facilities, they have elected not to do so. Of the 5,412 short-term general and other special hospitals in the United States, only 643, or 11.9 percent, operate extended-care units.[4]

Size of hospital seems to make little difference. Except for hospitals under 50 beds which, in general, have fewer resources, and where the number of extended-care units is quite low, no more than 15 percent of hospitals in any of the various size categories offer extended care. An examination of where these hospitals are located and the range of differences on a state-by-state basis is interesting. None of Delaware's 13 not-for-profit general hospitals, and only 3.7 percent, or 17, of 464 Texas hospitals have extended-care facilities. Hawaii's 28 hospitals have the highest representation with 11 or 39.3 percent providig extended care.[5]

Another important service for long-term patients is home care. Hospitals, with so many essential manpower, supply and equipment resources at their disposal, are ideally suited to sponsor, organize and operate home-care departments. Even with Medicare, Medicaid and some Blue Cross financing, hospitals have shown little interest in providing care to patients at home. Of 5,412 short-term general and other special hospitals in the United States, only 344 or 6.4 percent have home-care departments.[6] While it is true that the presence of an organized home-care department is more apt to occur in a larger rather than a small hospital, four out of five hospitals in the largest size category with 500 beds or more do not offer home care as hospital service. As with extended care, the lack of interest in this area of programming is relatively consistent among hospital providers.

It is unfortunate that more general hospitals have not become interested in long-term care because the need for alternatives to inpatient care is so clear. Partial hospitalization with flexible hospital admissions, extended-care and home-care services should be available and accessible for appropriate referrals of the chronically ill. Most often a proprietary nursing home or intermediate-care facility remains the only choice that a family has for the long-term patient. The patient must then be admitted to a facility where quality may be questionable and services limited.

Except for chronically ill patients who are experiencing acute episodes of illness, long-term care, per se, is usually not hospital-associated. Community general hospitals and our teaching hospitals are geared and relate primarily to the acutely ill or those who are undergoing elective surgical procedures. The chronically ill admitted to such places as psychiatric facilities, skilled nursing homes, intermediate-care facilities and rehabilitation centers are kept out of the mainstream of medicine. They are institutionalized in facilities lacking the benefits of highly organized medical staffs and modern biomedical equipment as well as the skills of many talented nursing, technical and ancillary personnel that are common to all good hospitals. Community general hospitals and those who are associated with them are preoccupied with patients who for the most part are admitted and discharged within a week or ten days.

It would be very naïve for anyone to assure that, even with complete involvement of the hospital community in the provisions of long-term care, most of the problems associated with providing health services to the chronically ill would be resolved. These issues are multifaceted, highly complex and broadly inclusive of medical, social, economic, political and attitudinal elements. There is little doubt, however, that long-term care services can be upgraded under auspices of community general hospitals with demonstrably high standards operating within a not-for-profit setting.

Hospitals have not become interested in providing long-term care for many reasons. They are strongly influenced by their own medical staffs, whose practices are individualized and highly varied. In general, however, most emphasis is placed upon the acutely ill patient and the often striking successes achieved in coping with crises occurring at the hospital. Experience in many areas has been good and results have been rewarding especially in the development of recovery rooms, coronary care, intensive care, respiratory, dialysis and other special units and services. Great progress has been made in applying knowledge and new skills throughout the major and subspecialty departments. Performances have been good and hospitals have been informing the public of many improvements in the management of patients who present high medical or surgical risks, and of better care now being received by premature infants, high-risk mothers and cardiac-arrest victims. Recently, hospitals have been reaching outside their own premises via mobile life-support units aboard ambulances with special equipment, radio-communication linkages and highly trained paramedical technicians so that myocardial infarct and other critically ill or injured patients can be treated en route to the hospital with the hospital emergency unit serving as a base from which instructions and orders are given prior to the patient's arrival. Most of this activity is dramatic, requiring crisis intervention; all of it is short-term.

The chronically ill patient, whose needs and problems are different and ongoing, is usually outside the hospital orbit. Admitted to a nursing home facility, the patient—most likely a female—is apt to be old, if not very old. She will have multiple diagnoses, impairments and a variety of social problems that are concomitants of her illness and aging process. She is apt to be widowed, living alone, and may have outlived her children. If she does have living offspring, they may be many miles away, living and working in other locations. She may not be able to walk without assistance and is quite likely to have mental impairment. She will be on multiple medications, taking four or more different prescription drugs per day. She will probably have some degree of cardiovascular disease, she may be senile, have suffered some kind of fracture and have arthritis. In addition she will probably be at the poverty or near-poverty level. This general picture is well-known to those in the health field, and the outlook for many of these individuals does not present any great hope for the future, given limited resources.

Irrespective of the difficulties to be encountered in any attempt to cope with the many problems of the long-term ill, we can do a much better job than is now being done. Hospital leaders and physicians must recognize and acknowledge our failures and omissions in this area. Better organization and active involvement of our community hospitals in the provision of long-term care and home-care services is strongly indicated in the face of the notorious Medicaid scandals within the nursing-home industry and the lack of high-quality care in many institutions. The federal government has failed to delineate a public policy for the long-term ill; our medical schools virtually ignore the matter when they should be pressing Congress and the Administration to identify and publicize a public policy; meanwhile, our hospitals are in default by concerning themselves almost exclusively with the short-term ill, whom they serve only briefly, episodically and discontinuously.

Hospital strategies may change, however, as a result of external pressures that all are undergoing at this time. Recent utilization review requirements at federal and state levels may cause hospitals to reconsider their priorities as demands for beds decline with implementation of externally mandated controls. These controls, which require continuous monitoring to guarantee compliance, have already shortened the average length of stay in many hospitals, with accompanying reductions in occupancy and revenue. When revenues drop substantially, some units may have to be darkened. In extreme cases, there may be mergers, acquisitions or actual hospital closings.

Hospitals which are in jeopardy because of low occupancy always consider long-term care as an option when strategies have to be changed. Converting an existing medical-surgical unit into a skilled or intermediate-care nursing unit may not be too difficult or costly to meet the long-run objectives of the hospital as matched against needs of the community. For hospitals with very high utilization and occasionally long waiting lists, the addition of a skilled nursing unit makes even more sense. For example, Norris reports very favorable experiences at Baltimore City Hospital, where the mean length of acute hospital stay for long-term care patients was 24 days less than that recorded in other acute general hospitals from which long-term patients were transferred to the chronic hospital facility operated by the parent Baltimore City Hospital.[7]

An important part of the concept of having skilled and intermediate-care nursing facilities and services under auspices of not-for-profit acute general hospitals is the thought that a hospital-operated home-care department should be integrated with the other activities of the parent organization. About 4 percent of all discharges from general hospitals are appropriate candidates for care at home. The majority of these are over 65 years of age, with the widely variable social, psychological, economic and health problems and characteristics of the elderly ill. Since one-half of all counties in the United States had no home health agencies in 1974, the need is obvious. It becomes even clearer in the light of the increasing over-65 segment of our population, which is now 21.8 million and which will have reached 23.8 million by 1980.[9] About 2 percent of the over-65 are bedfast and an estimated 6 percent are housebound.[10] The extent of unmet need for home health and related services among these 1⅓ million persons is great.

CONCLUSION

A clear national policy must be established to give direction and lend cohesion to the uncoordinated, uncommunicated and highly proliferated efforts and expenditures of billions of dollars in behalf of the chronically ill. In its absence, the American Hospital Association and the many state hospital councils along with counterpart representation at the American Medical Association and state medical societies should lobby vigorously for such a policy. This can be done through effors directed at our senators and representatives as well as pressure aimed at the Department of Health, Education and Welfare through regional and state health planning councils now being established with implementation of Public Law 93-641, the National Health Planning Resources and Development Act of 1974.

The federal government, in addition to establishing a national health policy for the long-term ill, must prescribe and enforce standards that will improve the quality of life and service within our long-term care facilities. The states have been inconsistent and have failed to do the job. More hospitals should become involved in long-term care, and hospital leaders—in partnership with their colleagues in medicine, nursing and social services—must do whatever is necessary to get more hospitals to develop programs for the long-term ill.

The federal government and hospitals are only part of the picture. A pluralistic approach is needed, and all agencies that are providing necessary services at reasonable levels of quality and cost should be reassessed, and Medicaid needs to be completely overhauled or discontinued. With national health insurance soon to become a reality, those who are interested in the care of the chronically ill must make sure that this group is not overlooked and rejected as they have been in the past. The long-term care gap must be closed. Now is the time to get started toward that end.

References

1. *Health Is a Community Affair*, Report of the National Commission on Community Health Services. Cambridge, Mass.: Harvard University Press, 1966, p. 103.
2. *Ibid.*
3. *Nursing Home Care in the United States: Failure in Public Policy*, Introductory Report of the Subcommittee on Long-Term Care of the Special Committee on Aging. United States Senate, U.S. Government Printing Office, December 1974.
4. *Hospital Statistics*, 1974 edition; 1973 data from *American Hospital Association Annual Survey*, Table 12B, p. 212.
5. *Ibid.*, Table 12B, p. 211.
6. *Ibid.*, Table 12A, p. 208.
7. Norris, John R., *The Acute Hospital-Chronic Hospital Affiliation: A Comparison of Length of Stay of Chronic Patients in Affiliated and Non-Affiliated Acute Hospitals. Medical Care*, November–December 1971, Vol. IX, No. 6, p. 483.
8. Report from American Hospital Association's Committee on Home Care to Health Insurance Benefits Advisory Council, 1974.
9. *Statistical Bulletin*, Metropolitan Life Insurance Company, November 1974.
10. Shanas, E., *Health Status of Older People. American Journal of Public Health*, March 1974, Vol. 64, No. 3, p. 262.

CHAPTER 2

MANAGEMENT

Management is perhaps the most valuable resource of a society. The theory and practice of management are now entering a stage in which the field has truly become an interdisciplinary area of knowledge. The evolution of management has occurred during the last century along five different schools of management thought.* They are: (1) scientific management, (2) administrative management, (3) human relations management, (4) behavioral sciences, and (5) management sciences. The integrating features in these schools are scientific thought, human orientation, and systems approach. The important concept for the administrator of long-term care institutions to grasp is that management is not a fragmented field of study. It is, instead, a fully integrated area based upon such disciplines as economics, sociology, psychology, statistics, and mathematics.

---

*For a detailed discussion see, Levey and Loomba (1973), and Loomba (1976).

Business organizations, private enterprises, and government can all be viewed as subsystems that are vital components in a society that is a large and complex system. It is important for managers to understand various conceptions of the fundamental relationships between individual managerial units and their host environments. Understanding the intricacies of these relationships is especially important for long-term care administrators, since their managerial units are extremely sensitive to societal values that define the host environment. PRESTON and POST (Selection 4) describe these relationships in terms of *social, legal, market contract, exploitation, technostructure*, and *interpenetrating systems* models. The main elements of each of the models are presented. These models can be very useful in describing and contrasting critical viewpoints regarding the foundations and nature of business enterprises.

KOONTZ and BRADSPIES (Selection 5) compare the "feedback" control system with the "feedforward" control system and emphasize the importance of the latter in management. Most reports are "feedback" control systems that merely inform the manager regarding what has already happened, and they are really post-mortems of what previously transpired. In a feedback system, corrections of outputs are fed back into the process, while in a feedforward system undesired variations of inputs are fed into the input stream for correction or into the process *before* outputs occur. The authors note that to achieve more effective control, it is necessary to reduce the magnitude of errors in reporting systems. Deviations should therefore be anticipated to avoid problems in the response time of a feedback system. The answer, therefore, is to monitor the critical inputs to programs. If changes in inputs are monitored, one can determine whether these would eventually cause failure to achieve desired goals.

The principles of feedforward control, used in systems engineering is an effective approach to managerial control. Any control technique involves the same basic process: (1) standards must exist; (2) the logic of control requires measurement of performance against standards; and (3) the process calls for taking action to correct deviations from plans. But the authors note that control is not this simple in practice and that control would be more effective if it were of the cybernetic variety. That is, its basic features should include "anticipatory feedback" as in a cybernetic system. Various techniques for future-directed control, such as cash forecasting, PERT networks, and related feedforward systems, are discussed. Guidelines for feedforward control are provided in the conclusion of the article.

BARNARD (Selection 6) describes an organization as a system of cooperative human activities, the functions of which are (1) the creation, (2) the transformation, and (3) the exchange of utilities. Four different kinds of economies can be distinguished from the viewpoint of creating, transforming, and exchanging utilities. They are: (a) a material economy, (b) a social economy, (c) the individual economies, and (d) the organization economies. The nature of these economies is described. The executive process, or process of organization, is the device for integrating different parts of the organization. The executive functions (communications, securing of resources, coordination, etc.) are part of the executive process. An important part of the executive (or managerial) process is to find an effective balance between the local and broad considerations, between the specific and general requirements. Barnard views the executive process as an art, rather than as a science. The terms pertinent to the executive process are "feeling," "judgment," "sense," "proportion," "balance," and "appropriateness." This description, in our opinion, is particularly applicable to long-term care administration.

Models of Management and Society

L. PRESTON AND J. POST

In the preceding chapter we referred to managerial organizations as microunits or subsystems within a larger society, and to society as a whole as a large and complex macro-system, containing numerous components and subsystems within it. In this chapter we extend these references to systems theory in order to describe and contrast some fundamental conceptions of the functional relationship between individual managerial units and their host environment.

We refer to these conceptions as "models" because they are highly simplified and brief sketches of very complex and even obscure relationships; yet such models can be useful as means of describing and contrasting critical viewpoints. For example, if one thinks of the private business enterprise primarily in terms of a *legal* model of the firm, certain basic characteristics, limitations, and roles immediately come to mind. If one thinks of it primarily in *economic* terms, another group of features is suggested. And when the firm is viewed as a *social* institution, still another set of relationships becomes paramount. No one of these conceptions is necessarily more complete or correct that another; and none of them *alone* provides a comprehensive basis for the analysis. Yet each

FROM: *Private Management and Public Policy*, Englewood Cliffs, N.J.: Prentice-Hall, Inc., 1975, pp. 14-28.

may be appropriately used for certain purposes, without reference to the others, and all may be combined if a comprehensive analysis is required.

Our analysis begins with a presentation of the *legal model* of the private business organization within our society. This conception is of intrinsic importance; moreover, it emphasizes the fact that the fundamental existence of managerial units as we know them rests upon their acceptance by society and, in the case of corporations, their specific authorization in public policy. The remainder of the chapter presents several fundamental and sharply contrasting conceptual models in which the legal, economic, and social characteristics of micro-units are combined and emphasized in various ways. The *market contract model*, familiar from traditional economic and political theory, is contrasted with its classic opposite, the Marxian model of *exploitation*. These two historic conceptions—which, upon examination, turn out to have some important features in common—are shown to be quite distinct in both assumptions and implications from the now-popular idea of a "managed society," as suggested by the *technostructure model* based on the analyses of Burnham and Galbraith. Finally, elements from these several prior models are *combined* into our own synthetic model, which is based on the concept of *interpenetrating systems*.

MODELS OF SOCIAL SYSTEMS

A *system* consists of two or more components or subsystems that interact with each other and that are separated from their larger environment by a boundary. *Systems* that are completely self-contained, involving no interactions with the environment, are described as "closed." Although a pure closed system is only a theoretical possibility, the degree to which a system is closed or open provides an important basis for analysis. Any "open" system—which includes any system that can be actually observed—is involved in some sort of transformation of inputs received from the larger environment into outputs discharged into that environment. The boundary of the system filters the type or kinds of inputs that the system can receive from the environment and the outputs that can be discharged. The boundary also determines the time rate of flow of input and output between the system and its environment. This general system conception is, of course, now widely used throughout the physical, biological, and social sciences.[1]

---

[1]Classic references to general systems theory include: K.E. Boulding, "Toward A General Theory of Growth," *General Systems Yearbook I*. (1956), 66-75; E. Nagel, *The Structure of Science* (New York: Harcourt, Brace, 1961); L. Von Bertalanffy, "An Outline of General

Social systems are invariably "open" and involve the exchange of inputs and outputs with the larger environment. Some individual social systems may be extremely and continuously open—with many different types of inputs and outputs crossing their boundaries at all times—while others are relatively closed or only periodically engaged in interactions with the environment. A household of family members intimately involved in the life of its local community is an example of an extremely open micro-system, a small subsystem functioning within the larger social framework. The same family living in a remote location and with infrequent and highly specialized contacts with the outside world might constitute a system almost closed.

Large elements of the social environment—communities, industries, regions, and so on—and even society itself are described as macro-systems or *suprasystems*, involving numerous large and complex subsystems as internal components. Some macro-systems exist only through the independent interactions of their subsystem components and without any overall locus of direction or control. *Dominant suprasystems*, however, are those which, once developed, take on an independent existence and exert a degree of control over their internal components. The national economy of the United States is a suprasystem in which central control or dominance is almost entirely lacking; even the economy-wide impact of federal government activity is only one among many influences at work within the aggregate. By contrast, a centrally planned economy is a dominant suprasystem; the overall plan is used to guide the activities of the subsystem components. Our own federal government could also be described as a dominant suprasystem originally formed through the interaction of the component (subsystem) states.

Systems are said to be *interpenetrating* when more than one distinct system, neither totally contained by nor containing the other, is involved in a single event or process. As Parsons states: "Where it is necessary to speak of two or more analytically distinguishable relational systems as *both* constituting partial determinants of process in a concrete empirical system, we speak of the systems as *interpenetrating*."[2]

System Theory," *British Journal of Philosophical Science* (1950), I, 134-65; and L. Von Bertalanffy and A. Rappaport, eds., *The General Systems Yearbook* (Ann Arbor, Mich.: Society for General Systems Research, 1956), annual editions. Our own orientation and terminology is derived from F. Kenneth Berrien, *General and Social Systems* (New Brunswick, N.J.: Rutgers University Press, 1968).

[2]Talcott Parsons, "An Approach to Psychological Theory in Terms of the Theory of Action," in *Psychology: A Study of Science*, ed. Sigmund Koch (New York: McGraw-Hill Book Company, 1959), III, 612-711. Quote from p. 649; italics in original. See also Talcott Parons, "A Paradigm for the Analysis of Social Systems and Change," in *System, Change, and*

Our own analysis of the management-society relationship is cast in terms of this interpenetrating systems concept. Therefore, we wish to distinguish as sharply as possibly between an *interpenetrating systems model*, in which two separate systems determine a single process, and two more familiar conceptions: *collateral systems models*, in which two or more systems are engaged in transformation and exchange relationships with each other; and *suprasystems models*, in which the activities of subsystems and components are dominated by system-wide authority or influence. These three general classes of models are illustrated in Figure 2-1.

THE LEGAL MODEL

The legal framework of our society is a suprasystem in which the authority of the state is used to preserve a stable and harmonious social order. In some instances—as, for example, with respect to criminal activity—state authority is exercised directly. In others, however, the state merely maintains a system of guidelines and institutions (laws and courts) through which individual parties can engage in collateral interactions to preserve and pursue their own interests and resist the impositions of others.[3]

The status of a business enterprise within the legal framework is a fundamental aspect of its existence. In general, the establishment and growth of private firms has been encouraged by our legal system, although private operations have been prohibited in some areas (not only criminal activity, but also postal service and national defense). At the heart of the relationship between the business firm and the legal system is the concept of *legal entity*. An entity is anything that possesses the quality of oneness and may therefore be regarded as a single unit. A legal entity is any unit recognized in law as having the capacity to possess legal rights and to be subject to legal obligations.[4] A legal entity is thus

Conflict, ed. N.J. Demerath and Richard A Peterson (New York: The Free Press, 1967), pp. 189-212. For an interesting application of this concept, see Raymond G. Hunt and Ira S. Rubin, "Approaches to Managerial Control in Interpenetrating Systems: The Case of Government-Industry Relations," *Academy of Management Journal*, XVI, No. 2 (1973), 296-311.

[3]See Harold J. Berman and William R. Greiner, *The Nature and Functions of Law*, 3rd ed. (Mineola, N.Y.: The Foundation Press, Inc., 1972), especially Chap. 1.

[4]Len Young Smith and G. Gale Roberson, *Business Law*, 3rd ed. (St. Paul, Minn.: West Publishing Company, 1971), p. 720.

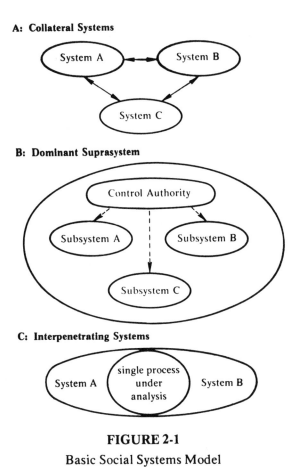

A: **Collateral Systems**

System A — System B

System C

B: **Dominant Suprasystem**

Control Authority

Subsystem A   Subsystem B

Subsystem C

C: **Interpenetrating Systems**

System A   single process under analysis   System B

FIGURE 2-1

Basic Social Systems Model

able to acquire, own, and dispose of property; it can enter contracts, commit wrongs, sue and be sued.

Human beings are legal entities of natural origin, possessing legal capacity and legal status. A proprietorship is such a natural person participating in market transactions as a business on a regular and continuing basis. A proprietorship is thus responsible for meeting all the obligations of a business firm, as well as those of an individual, as prescribed by law. Partnerships are associations of individuals participating in market transactions as a business on a regular and continuing basis. They are generally viewed as not having an independent legal existence apart from their members. Since a partnership is not a legal entity in itself, its obligations and responsibilities are those of the individual partners, each of whom—like the proprietor—is fully responsible both as an individual and as a business firm.

Although proprietorships and partnerships are much more numerous than corporations, the latter are clearly the dominant form of business unit in terms of economic influence. Corporations account for an overwhelming share of the revenues and assets of all business enterprises, and their pervasive importance in our society is even greater than simple numerical measures would indicate. However, each organizational form has certain particular advantages and disadvantages in specific situations; and once a legal form has been adopted by a firm, the form itself may have an important effect on the organization's capacity for and direction of future development. The essential feature of the *corporate form* is that it separates the existence and responsibilities of the organization from those of its individual human participants. Whereas the law simply recognizes and sanctions the existence and economic activity of individuals in the proprietorship and the partnership, the corporation exists as a creation of law.

The development of new forms of business organization and relationships has been described as an aspect of the enlargement of options available to individuals in the pursuit of their individually conceived purposes. Thus, the earlier common-law tradition of agreements and legal associations among individuals enforced by the judiciary gradually gave way to the development of collective organizations on the one hand and to an expanding role for the legislative arm of the state on the other. As Hurst comments: "It was inevitable that the legislature play a larger part in regard to corporation law. It did not lie in judicial power to grant charters, and men saw issues in this field too broad and turbulent to fit within the confines of lawsuits."[5] Thus, the state became the creator of new forms of organization, and widespread adoption of general incorporation statutes has greatly broadened the privilege of corporate form and served to popularize it.

The source of corporate existence is the *charter*. Unlike proprietorships and partnerships, which can arise without the formality of public approval, corporations cannot legally exist without governmental authorization. The chartering process serves to confirm publicly the view that the economic system and the organizations participating in it are performing a social function that is endorsed by society's political arm, the state. Corporate charters are either *restricted* or *general* in their terms. Restricted grants limit the types of activities that the corporation may perform. Thus, hospitals and schools, nonprofit

---

[5]James Willard Hurst, *Law and the Conditions of Freedom in the Nineteenth-Century United States* (Madison: University of Wisconsin Press, 1956), p. 15.

charities, and municipalities are each chartered to perform specific types of activities. Should the grants become outdated or merit modification, resort must be had to the public policy process in order to secure change. General grants, however, rely upon the larger system within which the chartered unit will be participating to stimulate the unit to act in a manner that will prove socially beneficial. General grants are, in effect, licenses for the corporation to act as its management sees fit, the assumption being that management's choice of activities will constitute a rational response to the stimuli generated by society as a whole and hence serve a "social purpose."

THE MARKET CONTRACT MODEL

The expectation that legal business entities will interact with each other so as to reveal and respond to social needs rests on an important historical idea that we shall term the *market contract model*. This model underlies the traditional doctrines of liberal economic and political theory. It is made explicit here so that the similarities and differences of other models to be presented can be clearly indicated and so that it can be referred to in later chapters, particularly in connection with the discussion of "fundamentalism" in Chapter 3.

The essential idea of the market contract model is that each participant in the economy—down to the individual firm, household, and productive worker—obtains its share of the benefits available in society by providing goods and performing services that are desired by other social entities and individuals. The firm or individual makes, in effect, a "market contract" with other members of society, provides them with something they desire on terms more favorable than they can obtain elsewhere, and obtains its own share of the "social product" from them in return. As Adam Smith described the situation: "Every man . . . lives by exchanging, or becomes in some measure a merchant, and the society itself grows to be what is properly called a commercial society."[6]

According to the market contract model, a business firm comes into being because it can perform desired functions for other members of society on favorable terms. If the market will sustain the enterprise, it continues and perhaps thrives. If tastes change, costs rise, or more favorable competitive alternatives appear, it declines and then must find some other functions to perform, or it will simply pass out of existence. Any problems that cannot be resolved by the market test

---

[6]Adam Smith, *The Wealth of Nations*, ed. Edwin Cannan (New York: Random House, Inc., 1937), p. 22.

must be referred elsewhere—to the political decision-making system, for example—or left to private social action and charity. Issues of "social involvement" are fully resolved by the basic test that some specific tasks must be performed on terms that at least some customers are willing to pay.

The pure market contract model is amoral and pragmatic, since, as Adam Smith pointed out: "It is not from the benevolence of the butcher, the brewer, or the baker, that we expect our dinner, but from their regard to their own interest. We address ourselves not to their humanity but to their self-love, and never talk to them of our own necessities but of their advantages. Nobody but a beggar chooses to depend chiefly upon the benevolence of his fellow citizens."[7]

The social philosophy associated with the market contract model is not, however, pessimistic or critical. On the contrary, the interplay of forces of self-interest is thought to lead as if by an "invisible hand" to a harmonious outcome for society as a whole. In the most idealistic version of the analysis, competition assures a close relationship between prices and costs; the accumulation of capital permits mechanization and the division of labor; and increasing productivity results in "the progress of opulence" over time.

Whether or not these conclusions can be fully anticipated, one key feature of the market contract model for present purposes is its assumption of a complete and sharp distinction between each market contracting unit, from the individual worker to the largest enterprise, and all other units and individuals within the system. It is a *collateral systems model* [see Figure 2-1(A)] in which each component entity is isolated from every other one, and interactions take place *only* by means of transactions. This assumed separation and isolation extends even to government itself, which, in the pure market contract analysis, is essentially a subsystem among other subsystems. It performs the key functions of maintaining law and order and providing public services, but its relationship with the other units of society comes down essentially to market exchange. Although Adam Smith himself, and most other writers in the liberal tradition, expressed strong personal views as to the proper (and improper) role of the political state, the model itself implies that the state should provide such services as the members of society desire, and on terms that they are willing to pay. Social decision making through the political process exists entirely apart from the market contracting system, and the latter is seen as the principal and most desirable form of social coordination and decision making. Any impact of government or other

---

[7]*Ibid.*, p. 14.

forms of collective social direction on the market contract process and its results can be unambiguously termed "interference."

THE EXPLOITATION MODEL

Diametrically opposed to the market contract model is a conception of the management-society relationship as a system of exploitation. Although this conception has its roots in the Marxian analysis of capitalist exploitation, it is equally applicable to the self-interested social dominance of dictators, commissars, and bureaucrats. (An old socialist joke has it that "Capitalism is the exploitation of man by man; socialism is the reverse.")

In the elementary Marxian exposition, capitalistic production inevitably involves the exploitation of labor by the capitalist (i.e., owner-manager) class. Marx viewed the value of all goods and services as due ultimately to the labor required to produce them. The capitalist hires labor and purchases materials in order to resell the resulting products at prices higher than costs, thus obtaining a profit. His object is not the production process itself (the production of commodities), but only the profit obtained (the production of capital). Each addition to capital increases the ability of the capitalist to employ labor and to expropriate additional "surplus value" (i.e., profit) arising as a result of production; and each round of production and sales increases the stock of capital and hence the capacity for exploitation by the capitalists. "Accumulate accumulate! That is Moses and the prophets!"[8]

The basic exploitation model was subsequently extended by Marx, and even more vigorously by Rosa Luxemburg, to include an emphasis on interracial and international relationships, particularly imperialism. "Capital, impelled to appropriate productive forces for purposes of exploitation, ransacks the whole world. . . ."[9] A half-century later an African representative to a conference on multinational corporations declared that a small nation is "virtually at the mercy" of such corporations in their "eminently rational" search for efficiency and profits. "No matter how one looks at it, foreign investment involves exploitation (in the Marxist sense) of the resources of the host country."[10]

In the modern version the *exploitation model* describes any situation

[8]Karl Marx, *Capital*, ed. Frederick Engels, trans. Samuel Moore and Edward Aveling (New York: Random House, Inc., 1906), p. 652 (This edition contains one volume only.)

[9]Rosa Luxemburg, *The Accumulation of Capital*, trans. Agnes Schwarzchild (New York: Monthly Review Press, 1964), p. 358.

[10]*Wall Street Journal*, January 29, 1973, p. 1.

in which a dominant social or economic class controls society for the pursuit of its own particular interests, extracting all available socio-economic benefits for use toward those ends. In this sense the exploitation model underlies the common conception of both the nineteenth-century "robber barons" in the U.S. and the political and administrative leaders in Nazi Germany and Stalinist Russia. It also accounts for the attitude, reflected above, of many less-developed host countries toward large international firms operating within their borders. The essential idea is that there are two types of collateral subsystems—exploiting units and exploited units—and that the exploiting units use their dominant power position to extract maximum benefits and thus maintain and enlarge their spheres of special interest.

The elementary Marxian notion of exploitation grew out of—and, indeed, in opposition to—the market contract notions of the classical economists, whose work Marx described as "learned disputation [about] how the booty pumped out of the labourer may be divided, with most advantage to accumulation, between the industrial capitalist and the rich idler. . . ."[11] However, the Marxian analysis shares with the earlier model a basic amorality. Marx viewed "the evolution of the economic formation of society . . . as a process of natural history," in which the individual cannot be held "responsible for relations whose creature he socially remains. . . ."[12] The notion of "social responsibility" (or irresponsibility) as an aspect of private business management would have been as foreign to Marx as to Adam Smith.

In all other respects, however, the Marxian model presents the sharpest possible contrast to the liberal conception of a harmonious society based upon market contract relationship. Where Smith and liberal economists down to the present—viewed business profits as essentially rewards for successful accomplishment of socially desired tasks and indicators of direction for needed economic expansion, for Marx the rate of profit was synonymous with "the intensity of exploitation." This reversal of relationships replaced the inherent harmony of the classical conception with a system of inherent conflicts and contradictions leading to ultimate collapse. According to the idealized market contract model, an entire economy in which each individual and organization operates on the same (i.e., market contract) economic principle is viable and stable. By contrast, the Marxian model identifies two distinct groups—the exploiters and the exploited—and holds that "capitalism . . . depends in all respects on non-capitalist strata and social organizations existing

---

[11]Marx, *Capital*, p. 653.
[12]*Ibid.*, p. 15.

side by side with it."[13] The capitalist system eventually collapses either because all possible exploitation possibilities are used up or because political and social revolution is brought about by the exploited groups themselves.

THE TECHNOSTRUCTURE MODEL

The market contract and exploitation models of the management-society relationship share a second characteristic in addition to the absence of moral and ethical content: They assume a clear and sharp separation between the ownership-control element of each individual managerial unit and the "rest of society" within which that unit operates. For Adam Smith, each economic unit, including the household, exists in isolation and relates to the rest of society through the mechanism of market exchange. Similarly, for Marx, each capitalist unit—and the capitalist class as a whole—is sharply distinguished from the rest of society and relates to it through the process of exploitation.

Both of these collateral systems models contrast sharply with supra-systems models in which society as a whole is shown to be functionally integrated and managed by some dominant control authority or group [see Figure (B)]. Centralized control by the state would, of course, constitute one form of suprasystem dominance. However, since there seems to be no widespread opinion that such a model would describe our current society, it does not require development here. On the other hand, the new-popular conception of an integrated society consisting primarily of large managerial organizations and dominated by their collective staffs of high-level professionals is a suprasystem model of some significance. Borrowing Galbraith's term, we refer to this conception as the *technostructure model*.

The technostructure model was first developed in Burnham's *The Managerial Revolution* (1941), and was more recently presented in Galbraith's *The New Industrial State* (1967). Both of these authors started with the familiar idea of the separation of ownership and control in the large business enterprise and the associated development of a professional managerial class. They then argued that the elite of the managerial class, whom Galbraith termed "the Technostructure," not only take over individual organizations within society, but these large organizations simultaneously expand and develop interconnections so that the techno-structure gradually comes to dominate society as a whole. This domination, however, is not essentially exploitative; neither can it be described in market contract terms. On the contrary, in the process of taking over

---

[13]Luxemburg, *The Accumulation of Capital*, p. 365.

society, the technostructure comes to be taken over *by* society, embracing social goals and objectives even as it shapes tastes and values through its own behavior. Eventually, the individual manager, the techno-structure as a group, the large organization, and society as a whole tend to merge into a single decision-action system in which particularistic goals, efforts, and rewards cannot be readily identified.

As Galbraith describes the process,

> The individual member of the Technostructure identifies himself with the goals of the mature corporation as, and because, the corporation identifies itself with goals which have, or appear to him to have, social purposes.

• • •

> It is the genius of the industrial system that it makes the goals that reflect its needs—efficient production of goods, a steady expansion in their output (and) . . . consumption, . . . technological change, autonomy for the technostructure, an adequate supply of trained and educated manpower—coordinate with social virtue and human enlightenment.

• • •

> Given the deep dependence of the industrial system on the state and . . . . its identification with public goals and the adaptation of these to its needs, the industrial system will not long be regarded as something apart from government. . . . Increasingly it will be recognized that the mature corporation, as it develops, becomes part of the larger administrative complex associated with the state. In time the line between the two will disappear. Men will look back in amusement at the pretense that once caused people to refer to General Dynamics and North American Aviation and AT&T as *private* business.[14]

The Galbraithian vision may yet be rather far from reality in the U.S., and its details correspondingly indistinct. By contrast, a similar technocrat-manager development has frequently been noted to be a characteristic

---

[14]John Kenneth Galbraith, *The New Industrial State* (Boston: Houghton Mifflin Company, 1967), pp. 166-343, and 393. See also James Burnham, *The Managerial Revolution* (New York: The John Day Company, Inc., 1941). The trend toward a managerial (rather than purely capitalist) society had been earlier detected by Marx, who should perhaps be viewed as the precursor of Berle and Means (*The Modern Corporation and Private Property*, 1973) as well as Burnham and Galbraith. Citing a now-forgotten "Mr. Ure," Marx states that "the industrial managers, and not the industrial capitalists, are 'the soul of our industrial system' . . . The labour of superintendence, entirely separated from the ownership of capital, walks the streets. . . . It is private production without the control of private property." Karl Marx and Friedrich Engels, *Capital*, III. (Chicago: Charles H. Kerr & Company, 1906), pp. 454-5.

feature of present-day Japan. "Japan Incorporated" has gained unques-
tioned use as a "description of one of the world's largest economies as
though it were a single, coordinated, centrally managed business unit. . . .
This relationship is not comparable to that of a socialist economy, with
the state in control . . . nor yet analogous to the United States in the late
nineteenth century, with government essentially an instrumentality of
big business."[15] On the contrary, the similarity of personal goals,
training, and experience among Japanese political, economic, and social
leaders apparently accounts for the overall harmony and broad social
comprehensiveness of their viewpoints.

AN INTERPENETRATING SYSTEMS MODEL

The two classic models of market contract and exploitation contain
several important truths. One is that the managerial unit is, to some
extent, a distinct element within society, not simply an operating
mechanism within some larger rationalized and controlled system.
Another is that there are elements of *quid pro quo* (exchange), as well
as elements of power and advantage (exploitation), in most important
social relationships. At the same time, the extreme separation of the
managerial unit from the "rest of society," whether for purposes of pure
exchange or unfettered exploitation, required in these models contrasts
too sharply with common experience reflecting cohesiveness and a broad
commonality of interest—and hence bases for cooperation rather than
conflict—along social entities. On the other hand, the full-blown technostructure model appears to overstate both the integration and the
rationality of social relationships and to underestimate the importance
of pluralism, adaptability, initiative, and innovation. Hence, we
present here a synthetic model, less precise than any of those previously
discussed, although admitting all of them—as well as many other
variations and combinations—as special cases.

Our model is based on the concept of *interpenetrating systems* [see
Figure 2-1(C)]. We assume that the larger society exists as a macro-
system, but that individual (and particularly *large*) micro-organizations

---

[15]James C. Abegglen, "Japan, Incorporated: Government and Business as Partners," in
Changing Market Systems . . . Consumer, Corporate and Government Interfaces, 1967
Winter Conference Proceedings Series, No. 26 (Washington, D.C.: American Marketing
Association, December 27-29, 1967), pp. 228-32. Quote from p. 228. See also Eugene J.
Kaplan, *Japan: The Government-Business Relationship* (Washington, D.C.: U.S. Depart-
ment of Commerce, February 1972). A sharp contrast is provided by the recent *America,
Inc.*, which takes an essentially exploitation-model view of business, political, and media
leadership in our own society. See Morton Mintz and Jerry S. Cohen, *America, Inc.* (New
York: Dial Press, 1971), paperback ed.

also constitute separable systems within themselves, neither completely controlling nor controlled by the social environment. As Cohen and Cyert describe the situation, "The organization and the environment are parts of a complex interactive system. The actions taken by the organization can have important effects on the environment, and, conversely, the outcomes of the actions of the organization are partially determined by events in the environment. These outcomes and the events that contribute to them have a major impact on the organization. Even if the organization does not respond to these events, significant changes in the organizational participants' goals and roles can occur."[16]

To illustrate the interpenetrating system concept, assume that some firm—an independent entrepreneur or one already organized—decides to pursue a particular path of technological research and development. The firm will draw information and resources—as well as ideas about commercially useful development paths—from the larger society. But the larger society will not in any concrete or conscious way control the development paths pursued—neither their direction nor their success. The development project may yield only trivial results, or none at all. On the other hand, it may yield an innovation comparable to the automobile, the computer, or the electric lamp. In the latter case, the firm does not simply "exchange" the resulting product in a collateral relationship with the rest of society—neither does it do so on a harmonious market contract basis nor in order to expropriate the surplus value. On the contrary, the introduction of the innovation by the micro-unit generates both new flows of activity and substantial structural changes within the macro-system itself. It is this ability of one system to change the *structure* of the other, and not simply to alter the volume or character of inputs and outputs, that distinguishes the interpenetrating systems model from simpler collateral or suprasystems conceptions.

The interpenetrating systems model also facilitates the analysis of the changing role of society, as expressed through formal public policy, *vis-à-vis* the managerial organization. In the market contract model, the state itself is merely one among many separate system units, collecting taxes and tolls in return for services rendered. However, the development of social concern for working conditions, culminating

---

[16]Kalman J. Cohen and Richard M. Cyert. "Strategy: Formulation, Implementation, and Monitoring," *The Journal of Business* XLVI, No. 3 (1973), 352. See also, Paul R. Lawrence and Jay W. Lorsch, *Organization and Environment: Managing Differentiation and Integration* (Boston: Division of Research, Graduate School of Business Administration, Harvard University, 1967); Neil W. Chamberlain, *Enterprise and Environment* (New York: McGraw-Hill Book Company, 1968); and J. David Singer, *A General Taxonomy for Political Science* (New York: General Learning Press, 1971).

in public policy actions to limit the hours of work or provide protection for health and safety, cannot be described in market contract (still less in exploitation) terms. On the contrary, we require a model that permits society to influence and constrain—but not necessarily dominate or control—an area of activity formerly reserved to the firm exclusively. Similarly, attempts by individual organizations to affect the course of public policy—whether by bribery or persuasion—may be described as an expansion of managerial activity into the decision system of society at large. In neither example does one system necessarily come to control the other completely, even with respect to the specific matter involved and certainly not in *all* matters. Nor can the relationship between the systems be described in the simple terms of input-output or exchange. On the contrary, the concept of interpretation seems to be, if less precise, the more accurate general form of the relationship between micro-organizational management and its social environment.

An interpenetrating systems model opens up the possibility—which has, in fact, become a necessity—of considering the potential differences, conflicts, and compatabilities among the goals of micro-organizations and those of society at large. In both the market contract and exploitation models it is assumed that organizations are responsive to their own individual goals and that these goals are balanced (favorably or unfavorably) with those of other system components through the exchange process. In the fully developed technostructure model there can be no goal disharmony; the goals of the managerial class and those of industrial society as a whole have, through the process of adoption and adaptation, become the same. By contrast, the interpenetrating systems model can accommodate both the separateness and possible conflict of managerial and social goals on one hand and the process of managerial/societal goal adjustment on the other. Society may take into account and seek to influence the goals of the managerial units; and they, in turn, may take into account and seek to influence those of society at large. Neither are the two systems completely separate and independent nor does either control the other; their relationship is better described in terms of interpenetration. As Virgil B. Day, vice-president of General Electric, has remarked:

> The social and economic responsibilities of the corporation have been so broadened and interwoven in the public's expectations . . . that it no longer makes sense, if, indeed, it ever did, to talk as if they could be separated.[17]

---

[17]Virgil B. Day, "Management and Society: An Insider's View," *Management and Public Policy* (Proceedings of a Conference, School of Management, State University of New York at Buffalo, September 1971), pp. 155-75.

> . . . [E]very corporation has not only a legal charter, that is, the charter of public expectations of corporate performance. These expectations derive from the current set of social values and national goals; and, as these values and goals change so too will the social charter of the corporation.[18]

SUMMARY

This chapter began with the presentation of some basic terms and concepts from general systems theory that were then used to delineate five theoretical models of the relationship between business organizations and their social environment.

In the legal model the individual firm exists as a subsystem within the suprasystem of the legal framework of society. Legal entities, particularly corporations, exist specifically as a result of social decisions and public policy. The legal status of such units reflects a social acceptance of their basic purposes and functional roles. Once this status is accorded, their rights and responsibilities—and their range of discretionary behavior—are defined by the suprasystem itself.

The two comprehensive classic models of the relationship between micro-unit management and the social environment are based on the diametrically opposed concepts of market contract and exploitation. Both of these models may be visualized as collateral systems. They assume that there is a distinct separation between the individual managerial unit and the society in which it exists. This separation can be bridged by mutually satisfactory exchange relationships, as in the market contract model, or by the exploitation of disadvantaged groups for the benefit of an ownership-management class, as in the Marxian analysis. An alternative and newer conception, the technostructure model, assumes that the managerial class controls and is, in turn, controlled by society, so that no sharp separation or disharmony of interests can exist. In essence, society as a whole is "managed" by the technostructure, but the goals of the managers and of society as a whole have become identical.

Although each of these familiar conceptions captures certain key features of reality, each is deficient in certain respects as a basis for analysis and interpretation of our own society. Therefore, we have suggested a model of interpenetrating systems, which assumes neither complete integration nor complete separation between micro-managerial units and their larger host environment. This model permits the analysis

---

[18]Virgil B. Day, "Business Priorities in a Changing Environment," *Journal of General Management*, I, No. 1 (1973), p. 48.

of both conflict and harmony, and of structural adaptation of the two systems to each other over time. The interpenetrating systems model is the core concept of management-society relationships used throughout the remainder of the book and is integrated with a more comprehensive model of the public policy process . . .

5

Managing Through Feedforward Control

HAROLD KOONTZ AND
ROBERT W. BRADSPIES

Managers have long been frustrated by making the occasional discovery—*too late*—that actual accomplishments are missing desired goals. Anyone responsible for an enterprise or any department of it has suffered the discomfiture of realizing that typical control reports merely inform him what has already happened and that most control analyses are really post-mortems. It does, indeed, do little good to find out late in December that inventory levels were too high at the end of November because of something that happened weeks or months before. Nor is it helpful to learn that a program is behind schedule or incurring excessive costs because of past events.

Most current control systems rely on some form of feedback. Unfortunately, a feedback loop must sense some error or deviation from desired performance before it can initiate a correction. This is, of course, after the fact. Moreover, since correction takes some time to become effective, the deviation tends to persist. The costs incurred, in many cases, increase directly with the duration of the error.

For example, the costs of holding excessive inventory are proportional to the time the excess inventory is held. The time slippage in a program may continue until correction is applied, and the costs of making

FROM: *Business Horizons*, June 1972, pp. 25-36.

up for the time lost usually seem to rise at an increasing rate. It is not surprising, therefore, that most managers consider the problem of control to be one of early recognition of deviations so that correction can be applied promptly. Although many managers have solved this problem to some extent through careful planning, simulative techniques, and network systems of control (PERT/CPM), truly effective control has rarely been achieved.

To achieve more effective control, it is necessary to reduce the magnitude of the error. To avoid the problems inherent in the response time of a feedback system, deviations should be anticipated. The only way to do this, short of using a crystal ball, is to monitor the critical inputs to a program. If we watch changes in inputs, we can determine whether these would eventually cause failure to achieve desired goals. Time will then be available to take corrective action.

At first glance, it may seem that such a method would be difficult to use in practice. Fortunately, there is now available an approach to effective managerial control through adapting the principles of feedforward control. This form of control is increasingly being used in systems engineering.

THE PROCESS OF CONTROL

Although planning and control are closely related, most managers see planning as the selection of rational means of reaching them, and regard control as the measurement of activities accompanied by action to correct deviations from planned events. It may thus be perceived that the function of managerial control is to make sure that plans succeed.

It is obvious that any system of controls requires plans, and the more complete, integrated, and clear they are, the better control can be. This simple truth arises from the fact that there is no way one can know whether he is going where he wants to go—the task of control—unless he first knows where he wants to go—the task of planning.

Control also requires an organization structure that is complete, integrated, and clear. The purpose of control is to detect and correct deviations in events; this must necessarily be done through people responsible for them. It does little good for a manager to be aware of variances but not know where in the organization structure the responsibility for them lies.

Given these prerequisites, any type of control and any control technique fundamentally involves the same basic process. *First*, standards must exist. While an entire plan can be used as the standard of control, the inability to watch everything usually forces a manager to select relatively few critical points that will reasonably measure how planned accomplish-

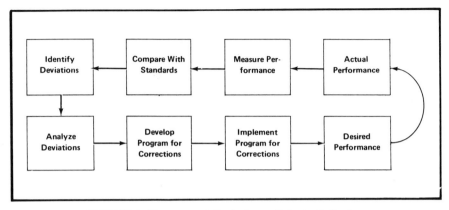

FIGURE 1. Management Control as a Cybernetic System

ments are proceeding. *Second*, the logic of control requires measurement of performance against standards. *Third*, the process calls for taking action to correct deviations from plans.

SHORTCOMINGS AND NEEDS

Control is really not this simple in practice, however, especially in management. Its basic features should be regarded as a cybernetic system as outlined in Figure 1. These steps represent the kind of feedback system that is involved in the simple room thermostat or the myriad of other control devices that one finds in mechanical and electrical control systems. But it dramatizes what every manager knows so well and many feedback engineers do not consider when they attempt to apply their thinking to management problems.

Simple feedback is not enough. Even the much-heralded ability of electronic data processing specialists to furnish information in real time, that is, as events are happening, is seldom good enough for management control. The fastest possible information may measure actual performance, may often be able to compare this measurement against standards, and may even be able to identify deviations. But analysis of deviations and the development and implementation of programs for correction normally takes weeks or months, if the correction can be made at all. Moreover, during this time lag, variances often continue to grow.

An inventory above desired levels may take months to analyze and correct. A cost overrun on a project may not even be correctible. A delay in an aspect of engineering or production, if recoverable at all, may be remedied only by an expensive crash program. Feedback is not much more than a post-mortem, and no one has found a way to change the past.

NEED FOR FUTURE-DIRECTED CONTROL

Intelligent and alert managers have recognized that the only problems they can solve are those they see, and the only way they can exercise control effectively is to see the problems coming in time to do something about them. In 1956, the senior author of this article identified future-directed control as one of the major principles of managerial control: "Since the past cannot be changed, effective control should be aimed at preventing present and future deviations from plans."[1] At this time it was emphasized that control, like planning, must be forward-directed and that it is fallacious to regard planning as looking ahead and control as looking back.

The simple principle of future-directed control is largely disregarded in practice, mainly because managers have been so dependent on accounting and statistical data instead of forecasts of future events. They have been too preoccupied with decimal accuracy, which can only be attained—if at all—from history. In the absence of any means to look forward, reference to history, on the assumption that what is past is prologue, is admittedly better than not looking at all. But no manager attempting to do an adequate job of control should be satisfied with using historical records, adequate as they are for tax collection and reporting on stewardship of assets to stockholders.

As a matter of fact, Norbert Wiener, the father of cybernetics, recognized the deficiencies of common feedback. He pointed out that, where there are lags in a system, corrections (the "compensator") must predict, or anticipate, errors. Thus, what he referred to as "anticipatory feedback" is often needed, particularly in human and animal systems. However, judging by the slowness in developing future-directed controls or anticipatory feedback in management control systems, there is little evidence that this variation of feedback has had the impact on thinking and practice that might have been expected.

TECHNIQUES FOR FUTURE-DIRECTED CONTROL

Relatively few techniques of future-directed control have been devised. Perhaps the most widely used is the continual development and revision of various kinds of forecasts, utilizing current expectancies to

---

1. Harold Koontz, "A Preliminary Statement of Principles of Planning and Control," *Academy of Management Journal*, I (April, 1958), pp. 45-61.

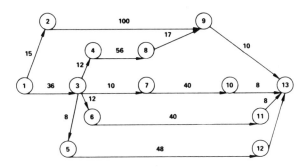

FIGURE 2. Simple PERT Network.*

*Circled numbers are measurable or verifiable events, and numbers of arrows are estimates of days required to complete an event.

forecast probable results, comparing these with performance desired, and then developing programs to avoid undesired forecast events. Many managers, for example, after realistically working out their sales forecasts may be disappointed with the anticipated results; they then may review their programs of product development or marketing to see where changes can be made.

Cash forecasts are also a widely employed kind of future-directed control. Because banks do not normally honor checks without funds in an account, companies seldom can risk waiting until late November to find out whether they had adequate bank balances for checks written in October; instead, they engage in future-directed control by assuring that cash balances will be adequate to absorb charges.

One of the best approaches to future-directed control in use today is the formalized technique of network planning, which is exemplified by PERT networks. In PERT/TIME the discrete events required to accomplish a given program result are depicted in network form (since few programs ever are linear in the sense that one portion of it is sequentially followed by another), and the time required to finish each event is contained in the network. As will be recalled, when this is done, the planner can determine which series of events will have the last slack time.

The simple PERT network shown in Figure 2 will illustrate this long-used technique and how the most critical path—the one with the least slack—can be identified. A major advantage of this tool is that, through careful planning and measurement of progress in each event, any time slippage becomes evident long before the program is finished. The time available to finish the remaining events is one of the inputs to those events; if it is less than the minimum desired time, steps can be taken to accelerate any event along the critical path that lends itself to speed-up at minimum cost.

If, for example, there is no slack time on the critical path of events "1-3-4-8-9-13" (in other words, if delivery has been promised in 131 days), the manager knows that if event "3" is ten days late the entire project will be late unless something is done now. Although PERT has tended to become so complex in practice that its use for actual managerial control has declined, it is basically the best single device of future-directed control that has yet been put into practice.

FEEDFORWARD IN ENGINEERING

As early as 1928, U.S. Patent No. 1,686,792 was issued to H.S. Black on a "Translating System," which incorporated the principle of feedforward control in engineering systems. However, the application of feedforward in electrical and process systems did not come into common use until a few years ago.[2]

In its essence, engineering feedforward control aims at meeting the problem of delay in feedback systems by monitoring inputs and predicting their effects on outcome variables. In doing so, action is taken, either automatically or by manipulation, to bring the system output into consonance with a desired standard before measurement of the output discloses deviation from standard. Thus, while feedback control relies on detecting errors in controlled variables as system outputs, feedforward is based on detecting and measuring system disturbances, and correcting for these before the system output change occurs. The basic concept of a feedforward and feedback system is outlined in Figure 3.

Feedforward has had wide application in the chemical and petroleum processing industries. It has been found particularly valuable where constant temperatures of material flow, exact mixtures, and various forms of chemical reactions require the precision that ordinary feedback, with its normal cycling, cannot achieve.

Perhaps the simplest form of feedforward control is contained in a

---

2. See, for example, L. F. Lind and J. C. C. Nelson, "Feed Forward: Concept in Control System Design," *Control & Instrumentation* (April, 1970), pp. 39-40; F. G. Shinskey, *Process Control Systems* (New York: McGraw-Hill Book Company, 1967), Chapter 8; F. G. Shinskey, "Feedforward Control of pH," *Instrumentation Technology* (June, 1968), pp.69ff.: J. A. Miller, P. W. Murrill, and C. L. Smith, "How to Apply Feedforward Control," *Hydrocarbon Processing* (July, 1959), pp. 165-72.

A review of engineering literature discloses a few references to feedforward control early in the 1960's, but the real volume of writing has occurred since 1967.

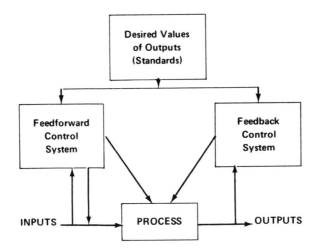

FIGURE 3. Comparison of Feedback and Feedforward Control Systems*

*In the feedback system, corrections of outputs are fed back into the process. In a feedforward system, undesired variations of inputs are fed into the input stream for correction or into the process before outputs occur.

system to maintain a fixed temperature of hot water leaving a heat exchanger where cool water inputs are heated by steam inputs. A thermostat on the water outlet would hardly be adequate, particularly with intermittent and variable uses of hot water; sudden changes in water output would probably cause bursts of cold water and steam inputs with resultant cycling of the water temperature.

To solve this problem, a systems design would provide a controller that would adjust the opening of the steam valve slightly. As the hot water usage starts to increase, the steam will be on its way into the tank before the water temperature drops below standard. A second feedforward loop might monitor the steam temperature and increase the rate of steam usage if its temperature should fall, in order to maintain the same heat input. By typing mathematical calculations into a computer that translates information to the input control valves, the oscillations characteristic of simple feedback systems can be reduced or entirely avoided.

However, even the most enthusiastic proponents of feedforward control admit that, if input variables are not known or unmeasurable, the system will not work. Therefore, for the best control, the use of feedback for output variables is also suggested.

FEEDFORWARD IN HUMAN SYSTEMS

The feedforward applications one finds in everyday life are far simpler than engineering applications. A motorist who wishes to maintain a certain speed does not usually wait until he notes that his speedometer has fallen below this speed as he goes up a hill. Instead, knowing that the incline represents a disturbing variable in the system of which he is a part, the driver is likely to start correcting for the expected decrease in speed by accelerating in advance.

Similarly, the average person does not wait until a rainstorm actually feeds back to him the need for an umbrella before he carries one. Nor would a successful hunter aim his gun directly at a flying bird; he would "lead" it to correct for the delay in his own system, his reactions, the gun, and the shot velocity.

It is, therefore, surprising that more thorough and conscious feedforward techniques have not been developed in management, particularly since the delay factors in ordinary feedback correction are so long. As mentioned previously in this article, this has been done by such means as forecasting end results and PERT/CPM networks. But a little analysis and ingenuity could result in much wider use of effective controls and even the future-directed controls now in existence could be greatly improved.

A number of illustrations of how the principles of feedforward might be used in management may be given. Many require development of mathematical models of the system so as to provide managers information of forthcoming trouble in time for correction, but space does not permit the display of such models here. The approach of feedforward can be shown by several simple schematic models. For this purpose, the cases of control of cash, inventories, and new product development will be presented.

Feedforward in Cash Planning

Since cash forecasting lies at the base of cash planning and control, this widely used technique of control is one of the best for revealing the application of feedforward to management. The basic inputs and construction of a cash control system may be seen in Figure 4. As can be noted, a number of input variables account for a desired future cash level. This model, representing a fairly simplified prototype of reality, shows that if any of the input variables differ from those premised when the cash plan was made, the desired cash level for the future will be affected.

As can be seen, many of these variables can have either a negative or positive effect on cash flow and the desired cash level at a given time in the future. It is readily apparent that normal feedback techniques are not

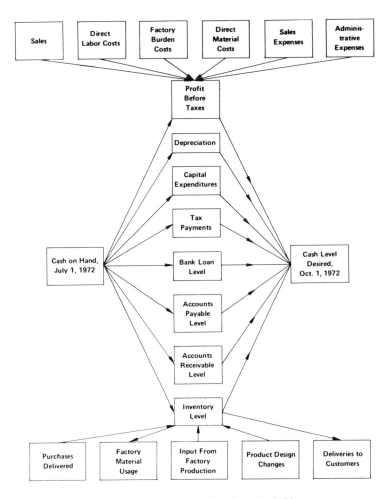

FIGURE 4. Input Variables for a Cash Plan

adequate, and constant monitoring of the various input variables, with a feedforward of their influence on cash, is necessary for careful cash control. Of course, one way to avoid the problem of shortages is to have available a ready bank line of credit. But what is likely to happen in this case is that the enterprise will keep unnecessarily high balances of cash, with resultant avoidable interest costs or loss in investment income.

It is also clear from cursory examination of this feedforward system that a mathematical model programmed to a computer can readily trace the influences of changes of input variables on cash flow and availability.

Neither this nor careful monitoring of input variables should be very difficult to do in practice.

Feedforward in Inventory Control

One of the most difficult problems in business is the proper control of inventories. Many enterprises incur large and often unexpected cost increases, as well as sizable demands for cash because of inadequate control of inventories. Moreover, as experience continually teaches us, an inventory discovered to be out of control on the high side is extremely difficult to get under control except, of course, through that most costly of all solutions—writing off excess stocks.

Also, the costs of carrying inventory, due to expenses from handling and storage, interest, property taxes, and possible obsolescence, are higher than generally assumed; 25 percent of inventory value per year is often regarded as a reasonable estimate. Nor should it be overlooked that inventory shortages often have high costs because of missed sales or lost customers.

In recent years, operations researchers have presented a vast array of mathematical inventory models and refinements. There can be no question that they have contributed greatly to effective planning and control of inventories, and many can be used as the basis for effective feedforward in inventory control. The difficulty with many models is that they tend to concentrate unduly on such matters as economic order quantities and safety stock levels. These may be appropriate for a mass production operation, but may not take into account the many other input variables, such as obsolescence or property taxes, that make effective inventory control so difficult and important.

Any company will do well to develop its own inventory model, using, of course, the many standard algorithms and techniques available, but taking into account as many as possible of the variables that may influence actual inventory accumulation.

The schematic diagram shown in Figure 5 reveals the complexity of inventory control. Once a desired inventory level is established in a way that minimizes costs in the light of demands for adequate inventory, the total (whether expressed in dollars or days of sales) tends to be used as a standard. Actual results are compared to it through feedback with little or no monitoring of the input variables on which the desired level was determined.

The attempt is normally made to maintain the inventory within desired limits by using only reorder point, economic order quantity, and maximum inventory level. In the simplest manual system, when a withdrawal is noted on a stock record, the balance is compared with the reorder

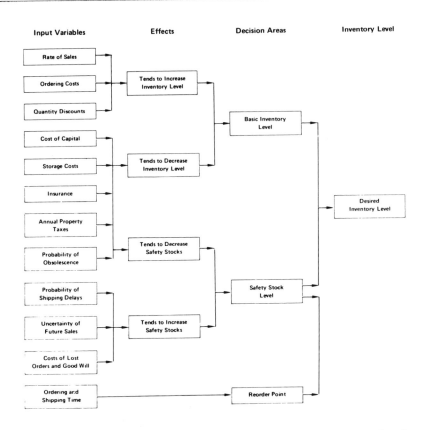

FIGURE 5. Effect of Input Variables on Determining Desired Inventory Level

quantity. When the balance on hand falls below this level a purchase order is issued. All of this may take place without considering the predictive changes of the original inputs.

The effect of such action may be to allow inventory to go out of control and raise costs. For example, if the rate of sales increased for a particular item, a company could find itself reordering too frequently or even running out of stock, thus increasing costs unnecessarily. Conversely, if sales decrease, a company could find that it was wasting cash by holding excess inventory. If sales declined further and a company continued reordering, it could find itself with a large obsolete stock.

If, instead, a company regularly monitored input variables, inventory levels could be adjusted by feedforward control by following the original decision paths and adjusting inventory purchases. In a company that used a manual inventory control system, for example, a simple monitoring

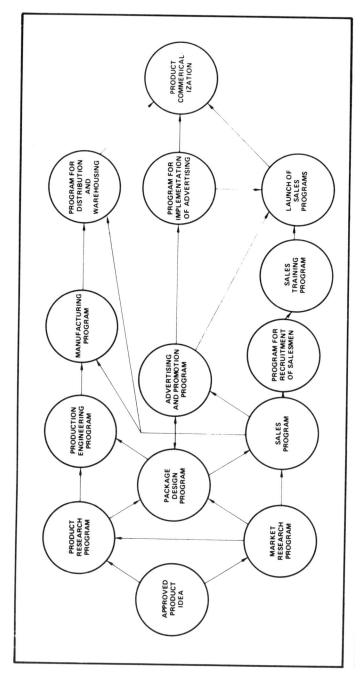

FIGURE 6. Feedforward Through a System of Interlocking Contributory Programs of a New Product Program

system could be devised. It need only consider significant changes in input.

However, it must be admitted that a more sophisticated computer-controlled inventory system would be able to adjust more accurately for the effects of smaller changes in input variables and thereby reduce over-all operating costs by keeping inventory under control.

In reviewing the various input variables, it can easily be seen that different departments within the company would have to be responsible for feeding information (probably into a central inventory planning and control unit) on the variables within its field of knowledge. For example, ordering costs, economic order quantity, and quantity discounts are usually best known by the purchasing department; shipping time and unscheduled delays in shipping are data that could be regularly expected from the traffic department.

Given a recognition of the types of input variables and a system for regularly collecting information on them, it should be easy to anticipate what is likely to happen in inventory. In feeding forward this information, it should be practicable to develop a kind of inventory control that is truly future directed.

Feedforward in New Product Development

The typical new product development program is, in the first instance, a system of interlocking contributory programs, as shown in Figure 6. It can be readily seen that this is similar to a PERT planning and control network. If times and costs are estimated for each program event in the network, the accomplishment of each subsidiary program becomes an input variable by which it is possible to feedforward the probable delays and costs of the completion of the program.

Moreover, each of the major programs in this network can be further broken down into a system of input variables so that completion of the total program can be forecast. Action can be taken in time to make necessary corrections and keep it under control. For example, within the product research program, there will normally be a number of subsidiary programs or events. These may include establishment of design definition and specifications; preliminary design of the product; development of a breadboard model; and testing the model.

Each of the other programs can be broken down into a number of subsidiary events or programs. These, in turn, constitute input variables to the individual programs necessary for the completion of a total product development program; their monitoring can feedforward both time and cost factors against the standards desired for the total program.

In addition, analysis can disclose a number of other possible, and usually unplanned, input variables that may affect a desired end result.

There are likely to be many of these, including such influences as delay in obtaining needed parts; failure of some part in a test; illness or departure of a key engineer; interference of a higher priority program; or change in a customer's desired specification. While not all of these can be carefully estimated in advance, and some may even be unforeseen, feedforward control can recognize the impact of such disturbances and provide for action in time to avoid program failure.

Change of Goals

In feedforward control systems in engineering, the systems are almost inevitably designed to correct input variables so that a given standard or goal may be achieved. In its application to managerial problems, the same approach can be used, but it should not be overlooked that the system may lead to changes in goals.

By placing emphasis on input variables, both those unforeseen, feedforward applications can furnish a means of regularly reviewing program goals themselves. A material change in interest rates, for example, may make a review of inventory goals desirable. Or a new development in product technology or market tastes may require a reevaluation of a product program. Managers must always keep in mind that goals and programs may become obsolete.

FEEDFORWARD CONTROL GUIDELINES

Although many other examples of application of feedforward to management control might be given, it is hoped that the transfer of engineering principles to management situations will be clear enough to help open the way toward the systematic application of feedforward in many areas. This can be done more easily than it may first appear. But in doing so several guidelines should be kept in mind.

1. *Thorough planning and analysis is required.* As in all instances of management control, thorough and careful planning is a primary prerequisite. But, especially in applying feedforward, this planning must be as thorough as feasible. Input variables should not only be identified but seen in their relationship and impact on desired end results.

2. *Careful discrimination must be applied in selecting input variables.* Since not all variables that *may* have some effect on output can be identified and monitored in typical management systems, it is essential that only the more critical variables be selected for watching. This is, of course, one of the key requirements of the managerial arena—to identify those elements that make a material difference in the operation of a plan.

3. *The feedforward system must be kept dynamic*. There is always the danger that input variables will be identified in the analysis stage and only these will be monitored. The alert manager will, of course, watch for new influences, either within or outside the control system, which might seriously effect a desired output. New technology, unexpected changes in loan rates and availability, changes in customer tastes, and even unanticipated changes in social or political pressures are examples of input variables that may not have been foreseen.

4. *A model of the control system should be developed*. Clearly, if a feedforward system is to be utilized, the area in which such control is desired must be defined, with the various significant input variables identified and their effects on desired goals analyzed.

This model may be a simple schematic drawing. It is far better, of course, to use an appropriate mathematical model that can be programmed in a computer. This way, the manager can take into account a larger number of input variables, more accurately calculate their impact on program goals, and be able more quickly and accurately to take corrective action.

5. *Data on input variables must be regularly collected*. Feedforward control is, of course, not possible without regular collection of pertinent data concerning the input variables so that the impact of this information can be carefully weighed. It is in this area that fast information availability is highly desirable and real-time information could have much meaning for control.

6. *Data on input variables must be regularly assessed*. No purpose can be served if input data are not regularly and carefully assessed to ascertain their influence on future program results. Barring unforeseen and unprogrammed variables, a computerized system can deliver this assessment quickly. However, for many feedforward systems the experienced eye and judgment of a top analyst may be good enough to point toward future deviations from planned results.

7. *Feedforward control requires action*. Few, if any, techniques or systems of management control are self-activating. All the system can do is to surface information that indicates future troubles, hopefully in time for something to be done to avoid them. This, of course, requires action. But if the system can be designed with enough lead time for a manager to take action, that is all that can be expected. And astute managers ask for nothing more than to be able to see their problems in time to do something about them.

There can be no doubt that feedforward is largely an attitude toward the analysis and solution of problems. It is the recognition that feedback information is just not adequate for management control and that a shift must be made away from emphasis on quickly available data on those input variables that lead to final results. It is a means of seeing problems as they develop and not looking back—always too late—to see why a planning target was missed.

6

The Executive Process

CHESTER I. BARNARD

The executive functions, which have been distinguished for purposes of exposition and which are the basis for much functional specialization in organizations, have no separate concrete existence.[1] They are parts or aspects of a process of organization as a whole. This process in the more complex organizations, and usually even in simple unit organizations, is made the subject of specialized responsibility of executives or leaders. The means utilized are to a considerable extent concrete acts logically determined; but the essential aspect of the process is the sensing of the organization as a whole and the total situation relevant to it. It transcends the capacity of merely intellectual methods, and the techniques of discriminating the factors of the situation. The terms pertinent to it are "feeling," "judgment," "sense," "proportion," "balance," "appropriateness." It is a

---

[1]The concrete phenomena are always acts or the effects of acts. Many acts appear so predominantly related to a particular function, however, that it is often convenient to think of function itself as concretely exemplified in an exclusive way. For example, an order appointing a person to a position may be considered exclusively the concrete expression of the function of maintaining the communication system of the organization. It will be evident, however, from the viewpoint of either origin or effect, that the act cannot be divorced from other elements or functions.

FROM: *The Functions of The Executive*, Cambridge, Massachusetts: Harvard University Press, 1966, pp. 235-246.

matter of art rather than science, and is aesthetic rather than logical. For this reason it is recognized rather than described and is known by its effects rather than by analysis. All that I can hope to do is to state why this is so rather than to specify of what the executive process consists.

I shall attempt this by presenting generally the sectors of the total action of organization in which the sense of the whole is the dominating basis for decision. To do so I assume that the reasons for existence, the ultimate purposes, are granted. The question then is whether these reasons can be justified by the results, whether the purposes can be carried out or attained. If so, it will be because the means employed are effective and because the action is efficient. Thus the two considerations to be taken into account from the viewpoint of the whole are the effectiveness and the efficiency of action.

I

It will be unnecessary for our main purpose, which is illustrative, to devote much space to effectiveness. It relates exclusively to the appropriateness of the means selected under the conditions as a whole for the accomplishment of the final objective. This is a matter of technology in a very broad sense of the term, including the technique of schemes of organization, of ritual, of technical systems, as well as the technologies of the applied sciences where they are pertinent. The non-executive view of these detailed technologies seems usually to be that they are technically isolated systems of production or of operation, which if significantly related in a particular cooperative system are so only in their economic aspects, or perhaps in ritualistic operations are related only in symbolic connections. In this view the breaking up of general purpose into detailed tasks involves the selection of a technology appropriate to each task, which may be treated by itself, independently of other technologies of the same coöperative system. What is then required for general effectiveness is only that the detailed technologies shall each be effective.

This is often true in a "practical" sense. In fact the incessant search for the strategic factors requires this emphasis. At a given time, for a given end, under given conditions, which specific technology is to be selected is the variable factor. We select which is the "better" method under the conditions which are granted. However, what must be emphasized here is that treating the total situation as a constant does not eliminate it, and that in fact there is a dependence of each technical process on all others used in the same coöperative system. The breaking up of general purpose into detailed objectives implies this. The precise form of the detailed objective is shaped by the general purpose and the possible process of accomplishing its fragments.

Clear illustrations of this fundamental integration of technologies as essential to the effectiveness of coöperative systems as wholes are easily available in many fields. To take one, the details of innumerable techniques of railroad operation are dominated by the single factor of the gauge of track. Another is the telephone instrument, the standard effectiveness of which, both for transmission and receiving, is the basis for limiting the variations of numerous quite different devices and structures under wide ranges of conditions. In these cases the word "standard"[2] is the expression of one of the concrete methods of insuring technological integration. Where this necessity is not obvious, it nevertheless exists. Disregard of it in principle is no doubt at the root of the incompetence and failure of many organizations. The principle is most significant in its bearing upon the size or the scope of coöperative systems. Much of the large-scale industrial integration of modern times may be ascribed to the necessity of controlling whole chains of technology as the means of effective accomplishment, quite aside from economic considerations. Conversely, the difficulty of avoiding the issue seems often to have meant uneconomic operation, that is, too large size has diminished flexibility and adaptability and compelled inefficiency.[3]

Thus the executive process, even when narrowed to the aspect of effectiveness of organization and the technologies of organization activity, is one of integration of the whole, of finding the effective balance between the local and the broad considerations, between the general and the specific requirements. As an analytically separable aspect of the executive process this field has been untouched by scientific inquiry, having been confused with economic aspects; but it has been considerably specialized in some organizations in the chief officers of their engineering departments, and so is specifically present in the actual conduct of much executive work.

Control from the view of the effectiveness of the whole organization is

---

[2]The word "standard" has both technological and economic implications. Sometimes it has direct social implications also. In the illustrations given it is the purely technological aspect which is in mind; but it is obvious in both cases that both economic (costs) and social (utility) considerations are involved. On the other hand, some standardization is primarily economic. One method is used not because it is necessarily the only one, or better than all others, but solely because economy results from the use of some *one* method.

[3]Note the inventiveness and innovations impliedly required in this situation. Technological invention is necessary to the accomplishment of many ends economically which can be accomplished, if economy is not required, by other means. On the other hand some ends which can only be accomplished by a given technological process cannot be economically accomplished without inventions and innovations in organization technique. The distinction seems generally not to be adequately understood. In consequence there is much fervent but indiscriminating discussion of the issues involved, in large- and small-scale production for example—or for that matter in large- and small-scale political or religious organizations.

never unimportant and is sometimes of critical importance; but it is in connection with efficiency, which in the last analysis embraces effectiveness, that the viewpoint of the whole is necessarily dominant. Under some simple conditions in small organizations this is a matter of common sense—for example, in the government of some small towns or the management of some small business. But often this is not the case. The common sense of the whole is not obvious, and in fact often is not effectively present. Control is dominated by a particular aspect—the economic, the political, the religious, the scientific, the technological, with the result that efficiency is not secured and failure ensures or perpetually threatens. No doubt the development of a crisis due to unbalanced treatment of all the factors is the occasion for corrective action on the part of executives who possess the art of sensing the whole. A formal and orderly conception of the whole is rarely present, perhaps even rarely possible, except to a few men of executive genius, or a few executive organizations the personnel of which is comprehensively sensitive and well integrated. Even the notion which is here in question seems rarely to be stressed either in practical or scientific studies. Any exposition of it must be an oversimplification and only suggestive. Patience is asked for the complexity of the following treatment because of the importance of the subject.[4]

---

[4]It has repeatedly been made evident to me by inquiring students that this subject is the most difficult so far as the approach to concrete situations is concerned, although intellectually it is grasped easily. Probably the reason is that a sense of a situation as a whole can usually only be acquired by intimate and habitual association with it, and involves many elements which either have not been or are not practically susceptible quickly to verbal expression by those who understand them. For example, I am asked to state to what extent and how economic facts and general economic knowledge govern my decisions in an organization. It is only with difficulty that I comprehend the question. It relates to a kind of world of which I have no experience—an economic world. I recognize economic aspects of my world, but I have to search diligently to find cases which seem exclusively economic. Let the reader take a balance sheet or an income statement—the most unequivocally economic statements I know of—and ask someone who understands those specific statements to explain them. Then observe how little of that explanation is economic except the money values that are assigned, and the arithmetical significance of these values.

All of our thinking about organized efforts tends to be fallacious by reason of what A. N. Whitehead calls "misplaced concreteness." Analysis and abstractions we must and do make in the most everyday conduct of our affairs; but when we mistake the elements for the concrete we destroy the usefulness of the analysis. Executive decisions are preceded by analysis as I have tried to show in Chapter XIV, but decision itself is synthetic. The background out of which strategic factors are analyzed is the whole situation to which the decision relates. This whole situation may be analyzed into physical, biological, social, psychological—and if you will—economic elements or factors, as I have incessantly emphasized; nevertheless the analysis is not the end but the beginning of purposive action.

II

It has already been stated[5] that the meaning of "efficiency" as applied to organization is the maintenance of an equilibrium of organization activities through the satisfaction of the motives of individuals sufficient to induce these activities. This equilibrium will be a resultant of several sets of factors. In principle a large number of specific combinations of these variable sets of factors could produce the same resultant.

I

An organization is a system of coöperative human activities the functions of which are (1) the creation, (2) the transformation, and (3) the exchange of utilities. It is able to accomplish these functions by creating a coöperative system, of which the organization is both a nucleus and a subsidiary system, which has also as components physical systems, personal systems (individuals and collections of individuals), and social systems (other organizations). Accordingly, from the viewpoint of the creation, transformation, and exchange of utilities, the coöperative system embraces four different kinds of economies which may be distinguished as (a) a material economy; (b) a social economy; (c) the individual economies; and (d) the organization economy. It is convenient for many purposes to abstract from these economies those elements which relate to exchange of utilities, as distinguished from the creation and transformation of utilities, under the name economics or political economy;[6] but we shall avoid doing so, so far as the limitations of language and the convenience of money measurements permit. We shall first discuss the chief considerations as to each of these economies.

(a) The material economy of a coöperative system is the aggregate of the utilities attached by an organization to physical things and forces which are controlled by the action of an organization. Two elements are involved in it: (1) the control; and (2) the assignment of the property of usefulness *by the organization* to these physical things. Both are necessary. Thus if it is believed that a piece of land would have utility if possessed or controlled by an organization, it nevertheless has no utility for the organization unless

---

[5]Chapter V, p. 56 ff. and Chapter VII, p. 92 ff.

[6]The thought here is that theoretical economics seems to cut across these four economies, as distinguished from an organization standpoint, including some parts of them and excluding others. In general, economics relates to those aspects that involve conscious exchange or that usually may be valued in terms of money of account.

controlled. Conversely, if a piece of land is so controlled, but ceases to be considered useful to the organization, its utility ceases.

The material economy of a coöperative system will be in continual change, because of changes in the physical factors and changes in the usefulness as determined by the organization economy.[7] These changes will come about by (1) independent variations in the physical factors—for example, the land may be ruined by a flooded river; (2) exchange of the *control* by the organization with individuals or other organizations, either for material or non-material utilities; (3) the depredations of hostile individuals or organizations; and (4) the acquiring of control by the creative act of organization—for example, the shaping of material into a tool. This latter is a form of conversion of non-material (biological and social) utilities into material utilities.

(*b*) The social economy consists of the organization's relationships (that is, power of exchanging utilities) with other organizations and with individuals *not* connected with the organization in a coöperative way, which relationships have utilities for the organization. It is the aggregate of the potentialities of coöperation with those outside the coöperative system.

The social economy is always changing. These changes result from changes (1) in the *attitudes* of external organizations and persons toward the organization or coöperative system because of *their* economies (affected by value attitudes, norms, institutions, physical conditions, etc.); (2) changes effected by exchanges of material or other utilities.

(*c*) The individual economy has been extensively discussed in Chapter XI. It consists on one side of the power of the individual, regarded here as inherent in or created by the individual, to do work (physical acts, attention, thought); and on the other of the utilities ascribed by him to (1) material satisfactions, (2) other satisfactions which we shall here call social satisfactions.

The economy of the individual is continually changing, because of (1) physiological needs, (2) exchanges made with others, (3) the creation of his own utilities, and (4) other changes in his state of mind, that is, his values or appraisal of utilities, physical and social.

(*d*) The organization economy is the pool of the utilities assigned by *it* to (1) the physical material it controls; (2) the social relations it controls; and (3) the personal activities it coordinates. It is the pool of values as assessed by the *organization* as a social system. It is the aggregate of the judgments or decisions as to the comparative utilities of non-comparable elements. The utility of a man's act is stated in terms of the utility of the work done;

---

[7]This does not exclude but includes, the usefulness that others give to it, *if the organization recognizes this* as giving opportunity for exchange.

the utility of the work done is appraised in terms of the things paid out to him. Thus the utility with which the organization economy is concerned is not personal evaluation, but *organization* evaluation in which the factors are (1) the factors of the physical environment, (2) the factors of the social environment, and (3) the factors of contribution and outgo from and to individuals. The appraisal of an organization is *not* a personal appraisal, nor, except incidentally, a market appraisal, nor the resultant of individual appraisals. It is and must be an appraisal based on its coördinative action—something unique to itself. It appraises physical possessions, social relations, personal contributions, on the basis of what it can do with them. It can create some utilities for itself by its action, it can gain some utilities by exchanges, it can trasmute or transfer utilities. Its ability to act depends upon the success of its action in maintaining the pool of utilities it can use.

The physical economy is the pool of physical things and forces controlled by the organization to which it ascribes utility. This pool may go up or down either because of external events or because of organization action; but the sum of the utilities ascribed to it may move similarly or contrariwise, and in disproportionate amounts. What determines the utilities is a set of circumstances not the same as those controlling the physical things themselves. The two sets of circumstances have in common some elements—the physical things. Other elements are diverse.

Similarly, the social economy is a pool of social relationships of the organization. Being immeasurable, they are difficult to state generally. They fluctuate, partly by reason of organization action, partly because of external events. They have utility for the organization, but the utilities change because of another set of circumstances.

Similarly, the individual economies or the aggregate of them change constantly partly by reason of organization action, partly because of external factors. But the utilities either of contributions from or expenditures to the individual economies will be dependent upon different sets of circumstances. It is hardly conceivable that the utility of a service should be the same thing to an individual and to the organization that uses it.

Therefore it is possible to analyze the status of a coöperative system from the point of view of any one of these economies. It can be stated what its physical possessions are, and in some sense (depending upon the criterion used), their economic value. It can be stated what the social *position* or assets of an organization are; and occasionally some kind of appraisal of the economic value is possible. It can be stated what the individual economies are in various sets of statistical enumeration—hours of labor, purchases made, wages paid, etc. It is often useful, and in many organizations necessary, to make such analyses or statements in terms of economics; and *parts only* of all of them are usually combined in balance sheets for commercial and most other organizations. *But the only statement of the organization economy is one that is in terms of success or failure; and the only analysis of that economy is the analysis of the decisions as to action of the organization. There is no unit of measurement for the economy of organization utility.*[8]

II

The equilibrium of the organization economy requires that it shall command and exchange sufficient of the utilities of various kinds so that it is able in turn to command and exchange the personal services of which it is constituted. It does this by securing through the application of these services the appropriate supplies of utilities which when distributed to the contributors ensure the continuance of appropriate contributions of utilities from them. Inasmuch as each of these contributors requires a surplus in *his* exchange, that is, a net inducement, the organization can survive only as it secures by exchange, transformation, and creation a surplus of utilites in its own economy. If its operations result in a deficit, it is less and less able to command the organization activities of which it consists. The organization must pay out material utilities and social utilities. It cannot pay out more than it has. To have enough it must secure them either by exchange or by creating them.

For illustration, take first a religious organization. It could not, in most cases, have command of a surplus of material utilities, yet it must have such utilities in order to pay them out to those who require them—principally clergymen and lay assistants of various kinds who devote most of their efforts to the church. Its supply of these utilities must therefore come from communicants (contributors), who may contribute little effort beyond attention, attendance at services, etc. For these material utilities it exchanges what we have called social utilities, which are partly a result of its ritual and community creations. This is in part a transformation of material utilities to social utilities. In order to do this it

---

[8]Compare, in this connection Pareto's distinction between the utility *of* a society and the utility *for* a society (*Sociologic Générale*, paragraphs 2128 ff.), also Talcott Parsons (*The Structure of Social Action*, pp. 241-249). I judge that what Pareto was talking about and what I am attempting to develop are equivalent in principle; but I am not certain. Using his phraseology I am saying that the aggregate of the utilities of the organization connection of each "member" of an organization is one economy and may be called the utility for an organization; but that there must be a utility *of* the organization which is based upon entirely different factors but includes the *individual* utilities. This utility *of* the organization is necessarily the social evaluation by the system of its own action and *cannot* be the sum of individual appraisals. In my phrase the utility *of* the organization is the organization economy, that is, *I* stress its incessantly dynamic character.

may have to expend both material utilities and social utilities in proselyting, which will result in additional contributors who increase either the surplus of physical or of social utilities. To do this it will pay material utilities to some (those who require them for direct or indirect missionary effort) and social utilities to others (those who possess "zeal" for the missionary cause). Thus in the organization economy the factors are interacting and interdependent.

For a second illustration, take a government. Even when not a creator or direct securer of physical utilities, it requires great quantities of them. It also requires social utilities in the form of support and acquiescence of organizations and individuals.

It will secure its physical utilities by taxes on individuals and organizations, but must also secure social contributions under the form of patriotism, willingness to be taxed, etc.

Take a third illustration, an industrial organization. It must produce physical utilities, for which purpose it is adapted, and must also distribute social utilities. If it can produce surpluses of physical utilities they can be used to some degree to secure social utilities for distribution, but some of the latter at least it must also create. If there is a scarcity of both, it may expend some of either to change a state of mind, reducing the necessity for the drain on its supplies of one or the other or both.

CHAPTER 3

VALUE SYSTEMS AND LONG-TERM CARE

Man has continuously attempted to conquer disease and increase his life span. The expected life span in the United States increased from 54 years in 1920 to 73 years in 1976. However, progress in extending life expectancies at age 65 has been limited by gaps in information regarding the aging process and methods of controlling it. Those individuals who reach the age of 65 can now expect to live an additional 14.8 years as compared to 10.8 years in 1900. That represents an increment of only 4.2 years over the last three quarters of a century. Greater expenditures for gerontological research will undoubtedly occur when break-throughs begin to emerge and when such expenditures are regarded as reasonably probable and socially desirable.

The proportion of aged citizens in the total population of the United States increased from 2.5 percent in 1850 to 9.9 percent in 1970. The greater number of aged, and associated chronic illness has resulted in a significant expansion of the long-term care industry, particularly in the last two decades. In spite of this rapid growth, the field of long-term care has been relegated to a marginal role in the health-care system. This peripheral position has evolved directly from the responses of society to the problems of the chronically ill and the aged. It appears that the preoccupation of society has been with growth, affluence, and the *quantitative* dimensions of life. However, it is increasingly recognized that it is the *quality* of life that matters. A respected old age and qualitative comforts seem to be among the key desires and objectives of most human beings. And these are the very factors that are largely determined by the value systems of society. These values, which are derived from our cultural heritage, are guides to social behavior, and they specify what society will do with our limited time and resources. It is unfortunate that we have not demanded high standards of long-term care, even though the expected norm in the acute-care sector is generally otherwise.

A number of factors account for the relative disinterest in long-term care on the part of society and its institutions. First is the often-cited orientation of American society to values that are associated with the preservation of youth. The elderly are not particularly respected as teachers and guardians of societal values, and the attitudes of the young toward this group are not indicative of respect for knowledge that comes with age and experience. Second, the aged as a group and institutionalized chronically ill patients do not yet possess a significant base of power and influence, in spite of the fact that they now constitute a sizable portion of the population. Third, the primary focus of educational institutions that are engaged in health training and research has been toward patients with acute-care problems, and the long-term care sector has received only sparse attention.

Long-term care services are not regarded as an especially high priority in terms of public expectations for better standards of care and more efficient methods of regulation. Only recently have nursing homes and mental hospitals received the attention of the media, and even this has usually resulted from such negative factors as financial scandals and patient abuse. Now, in the post-Medicare period, improvements in the regulation of long-tem care facilities are being made. However, much remains to be accomplished. In fact, the majority of long-term care institutions are oriented, because of rigidities of state and federal reimbursement policies, to merely operating at minimal levels of staffing and performance. While this situation may not be regarded as especially harmful for the majority of institutionalized patients, a significant number of patients do require special rehabilitative, social, and recreational services, and these are often entirely lacking or provided in a meager or haphazard fashion. Improvements will, above all, require a reorientation of our social values toward the aging and the chronically-ill.

It is important to recognize that values seldom function in a pure and abstract form. They influence, and in turn are influenced by, social environments and fiscal realities. Decisions based upon value judgments and value systems are part of our everyday lives. It is clear that what is valued in society is reflected in the structures, processes, and outcomes of our institutions and in the way people live together. Thus significant changes in institutional arrangements for long-term care services will be very gradual unless there are massive infusions of capital, or major breakthroughs in the control of the aging process. That is, without the technological breakthroughs or further major increases in gross national product, the existing state of affairs in long-term care institutions will not be greatly affected. And this can happen only if the society begins to place a major emphasis on long-term care.

Federal and state governments are the major purchasers of long-term care services. They remain the key, but thus far inadequate, source of economic support for long-term care. The picture can improve in one of two ways. First, sufficient public pressure must emerge in order to generate a change in the attitude of the federal and state governments. Second, the value judgments of society must create viable alternatives to institutional care. In any case, the future clearly requires the development of a comprehensive long-term care and geriatric services system.

KATZ and GEORGOPOULOS (Selection 7) note that organizations are being challenged as the result of a number of important factors, including the break with traditional authority patterns, the growth of democratic ideology, economic affluence and consequent changes in needs and motivations, and the accelerated rate of change. They indicate that adaptive sub-systems have not been able to keep pace with other organizational subsystems, and new inputs tend to be either spontaneously rejected or else incorporated without assimilation in the dominant patterns. The leadership in most organizations is preoccupied with the tasks of mediating between conflicting demands. Thus the reconceptualization of values has usually been in the hands of rebelling factions. The authors conclude that there is hope that a consensus may emerge, which recognizes that organizational restructuring is necessary and which acknowledges both the role of direct democracy in the smaller units and representative democracy in the larger system. It is important for the administrator of the long-term care facility to recognize that the extent of organizational restructuring and changes in corporate values must be in balance with professional roles and their recognition of patients' needs.

Long-term care administrators must be concerned with the impact of institutionalization upon the success of patient-care programs. LIEBERMAN (Selection 8) assesses current knowledge and research strategies regarding the effects of institutional environments on the elderly and attempts to provide a framework for future research efforts. Temporary institutionalization or settings which do not provide multiple centralized services are not included in the discussion. The author acknowledges that the common sense impression that institutions have negative effects on the psychological well-being and physical survival of aged adults appears to be supported by a number of empirical studies. Some investigators have reported marked increases in mortality rates for aged persons entering mental institutions or homes for the aged.

The studies referred to by the author clearly demonstrate that aged persons in institutions are likely to die sooner than aged persons in the general population and that the institutionalized aged are psychologically disadvantaged. The author cautions that institutionalization may not be the key variable in causing such differences, and he discusses evidence related to this issue. He examines the impact of changing the environment of elderly individuals, including the effect of the intra-institutional shifts and length of stay upon sample populations. The author concludes that the common stereotypes regarding the negative influences of institutionalization upon the aged have been overdrawn.

MORISON (Selection 9) notes that most people now die of

chronic illnesses and degeneration. Unfortunately both the public and the medical profession frequently hold attitudes that may not be conducive to assisting the aged patient to adapt to altered psychological and physiological circumstances. He emphasizes that technological progress has increased the number of "options" in therapy and that ultimately all methods of choice can be reduced to personal value judgments. Many of the treatment options are complex and are often painful and costly. Most therapeutic decisions for the aged are accordingly not "life-or-death decisions in any simple either-or sense." Judgments have to be made regarding the probable quality of life and time that is left to the patient.

Morison indicates that the medical profession has brought about much of the criticism that now surrounds it because it has failed to maintain a technological-humanitarian balance. However, the last few years have witnessed a considerable upsurge of interest in the problems of death and dying. Approaches to this topic may be separated into two areas: the first deals with making the last days of the individual as comfortable as possible and the second with the propriety of allowing or helping the individual to die at an appropriate time. The author discusses various alternatives to the nursing home such as the hospital and home care. He then moves to the very important issue of when it becomes appropriate to die and the complexities of definition and attitude that surround the subject. He concludes that changing attitudes to death and dying "provide an excellent paradigm of how changing technologies force on us the consideration of equally significant changes in value systems and social institutions."

7

Organizations in a Changing World

DANIEL KATZ
BASIL S. GEORGOPOULOS

Our nation has been aptly characterized as an *organizational society* (Presthus, 1962). Most of our working hours are spent in one organizational context or another. If the dominant institution of the feudal period was the church, of the early period of nationalism the political state, the dominant structure of our time is the organization. Even among those in revolt the old union line still works: "Organize the guys."

But organization forms today are under challenge and without creative modification may face difficulties in survival. On the one hand they are growing in size and complexity, with criss-crossing relationships with other systems and with increasing problems of coordination, integration, and adaptation. The traditional answer in organization structure is on the technical side, *more* computerized programs for feedback and coordination, *more* specialization of function, *more* centralization of control. Yet the social and psychological changes in the culture are increasingly at odds with the technological solution calling for more and more of the same. Technological efficiency far surpasses social efficiency in most cases, even though neither is a substitute for the other from the standpoint of organi-

---

FROM: *Journal of Applied Behavioral Science*, Vol. 7, May-June 1971, pp. 342-357.

zational effectiveness; and the gap is widening so as to generate serious conflict within the system.

Before exploring this conflict and its implications in greater detail, let us examine briefly the structure and functioning of organizations as open social systems. We can distinguish among the subsystems which comprise the larger structure (Katz & Kahn, 1966). The production, or instrumental, subsystem is concerned with the basic type of work that gets done, with the "throughput"—the modification of inputs which result in products or services. Attached to the productive subsystem are the supportive services of procurement of supplies material and resources, and the disposal of the outputs.

The maintenance, or social, subsystem is concerned not with the physical plant but with the social structure, so that the identity of the system in relation both to its basic objectives and the environment is preserved. People not only have to be attracted to the system and remain in it for some period of time but they have to function in roles which are essential to the mission of the organization. The maintenance subsystem is concerned with rewards and sanctions and with system norms and values that ensure the continuity of the role structure. In short, its function has to do with the psychological cement that holds the organizational structure together, with the integration of the individual into the system. The channeling of collective effort in reliable and predictable pathways is the basis of organizational structure.

✓ The managerial subsystem cuts across all other subsystems as a mechanism of control, coordination, and decision making and as a mechanism for integrating the instrumental and maintenance functions of the organization. To meet environmental changes both with respect to inputs and receptively for outputs and to handle system strains, the managerial subsystem develops adaptive structures of staff members as in the case of research, development, marketing, and planning operations.

Let us look at the maintenance function more closely, however, before considering the adaptation problem in the light of major societal changes. Over time it requires more than sheer police power and coercive sanctions. It depends upon some degree of integration or involvement of people in terms of their own needs. Values, norms, and roles tie people into the system at different psychological levels and in different ways (Parsons, 1960).

Values provide the deepest basis of commitment by their rational and moral statement of the goals of a group or system. To the extent that these values are accepted by individuals as their own beliefs, we speak of the internalization of group goals. The degree of internalization will vary among the members of any group, but it is important for all organizations to have some hard core of people dedicated to their mission both for accomplishment of many types of tasks and as models for others. Such value commitment can come about through self-selection into the system of those possessing beliefs congruent with its goals, through socialization in the general society or in the organization, and through participation in the rewards and decision making of the group. The internalization of group goals is facilitated by the perception of progress toward these objectives. Such progress is interpreted as an empirical validation of values.

Normative involvement refers to the acceptance of system requirements about specific forms of behavior. These requirements are seen as legitimate because rules are perceived as necessary and because in general the rules are equitable. A particular demand by a particular officer may be seen as unjust, but in general there is acceptance of the need for directives from those in positions of authority, provided that they have attained their positions properly and that they stay within their areas of jurisdiction in the exercise of their authority. In complex organizations, such as universities, hospitals, and industrial firms, the rules of the game can be improved, but they are universalistic and do not permit particularistic favoritism or discrimination.

At the level of *role behavior* people make the system function because of their interdependence with others, the rewards for performing their roles, and the socio-emotional satisfactions from being part of a role-interdependent group. In carrying out their roles, organizational members at all times but in varying degrees are interdependent both functionally and psychologically. Not all role performance provides expressive gratifications, however, and hence other rewards such as monetary incentives and opportunities for individual achievement, as well as group accomplishment and socio-emotional satisfactions, can be linked to adequate behavior in the given role. In most large organizations extrinsic rewards of pay, good working conditions, and so on are relied on heavily.

It is apparent that these three levels of member involvement are not necessarily intrinsically related. The values of a particular organization may have little to do with many of the roles in the system, and the norms of legitimacy are not necessarily specific to organizational values. A research organization may furnish a nice fit among values, norms, and roles for its research workers but a poor fit for its supportive personnel. Few organizations, however, can rely on value commitment alone to hold their members, and hence they maximize other conditions and rewards to compete with other systems. The development of universalistic norms under the impact of bureaucratic organization forms has provided great mobility for people in an expanding economic society, and thus has contributed to its growth—at the expense of value commitment.

In a well-integrated system, however, there is some relationship among these levels so that they are mutually reinforcing. In an ideal hospital, even the attendant can be affected by the values of saving lives and improving health, can perceive the normative requirements as necessary and fair, and derive satisfaction from his role, particularly if he is made part of a therapy team. Values can contribute to the strength of the normative system in providing a broader framework of justifiable beliefs about the rightness of given norms. Thus norms can be seen not only as equitable rules but as embodiments of justice and of equality. The strength of maintenance forces lies in the many mechanism for supporting the role structure and for some degree of mutual reinforcement.

The problem of how to organize human effort most effectively in complex, specialized organizations within a rapidly changing sociocultural environment, while maintaining the integrity of the system, is of utmost significance and concern everywhere in our time. Its solution generally demands greater social-psychological sophistication, however, rather than a more sophisticated work technology (Georgopoulos, 1970). It requires social organization innovations and the testing of new forms and patterns of organization, or at least significantly modified organizational structures than those now in operation (Georgopoulos, 1969; Likert, 1967). It will not be achieved at acceptable levels simply by an even more perfect technology at our disposal. As profound changes continue to occur in society at rapid but uneven rates, organizational viability and effectiveness are in jeopardy unless the social efficiency of the system can more clearly match its technological efficiency in the vast majority of organizations, and unless the adaptability of organizations can be improved well beyond current levels.

Four major changes have occurred in our society which challenge both the production and social subsystems of organizations: (a) a break, at first gradual and now pronounced, with traditional authority and the growth of democratic ideology; (b) economic growth and affluence; (c) the resultant changes in needs and motive patterns; and (d) the accelerated rate of change. These changes are significant for organizations, since as open systems organizations are in continuing interaction with their environment both with respect to production inputs of material resources and social inputs from the culture and from the larger social structure.

The break with the older pattern of authority has eroded some of the formerly dependable maintenance processes of organizations. Bureaucratic systems had long profited from the socialization practices of traditional society, in which values and legitimacy had a moral basis of an absolutist character. It was morally wrong to reject in word or deed the traditional teachings about American institutions. It was wrong to seek change other than through established channels. Not everyone, of course, lived up to the precepts, but deviance was easy to define and highly visible, and those who deviated generally felt guilty about their misconduct. If they did not, they were considered to be psychopaths. Organizations had the advantage of a degree of built-in conformity to their norms and in some cases to their values because of the general socialization in the society about agreed-on standards. This consensus, moreover, made nonconformity a matter of conscience. There was an all-or-none quality about virtue, honesty, and justice, and these values were not seen as relativistic or empirical generalizations. Member compliance with organizational norms and values no longer can be sustained on the basis of authority (Etzioni, 1964; Georgopoulos, 1966; Georgopoulos & Matejko, 1967).

The very growth of bureaucratic systems helped to demolish absolutist values of a moral character. As conscious attempts to organize collective enterprises, organizations were guided by rational objectives and empirical feedback. Pragmatism replaced tradition. Results and accomplishment were the criteria rather than internal moral principle. Furthermore, the normative system shifted, as Weber (1947) noted, from traditional authority to rational authority. Rules and laws were the instruments of men to achieve their purposes and lacked any transcendental quality. They could be changed at will as situations and needs changed or they become ineffective. Having undercut the traditional basis of authority, the bureaucratic system can no longer rely upon the older moral commitment to its directives.

The growth of organizations affected the larger society and its socialization practices and in turn was affected by it. The training of children in a rational and democratic framework further increased a nontraditional orientation to values and norms.

The decline of traditional authority has been accompanied by the growth of the Democratic Ethic and democratic practices. The source of power has been shifting from the heads of hierarchies and from oligarchies to the larger electorate. This process can be observed in the political system where restrictions have been removed on suffrage. Nonproperty owners, women, and now blacks are eligible to vote. Indirect mechanisms of control from above are changing as in the political conventions of major parties. Democratic ideas of governance have extended into other institutions as well.

The tremendous technological advances which have increased the productivity of the nation need no documentation. We are already using the phrase "postindustrial society" to characterize our era. This development raises questions about the basic functions of colleges and universities. Havighurst (1967) has pointed out that in the past, two functions have been dominant: the *opportunity function* and the *production function*. Education was a means of social mobility, the opportunity function. On the production side, education provided the training for professional, technical, and industrial roles in the society. Today, however, when we are over the economic hump, these two functions are less important and a third function comes to the fore: the *consumption function*. "Education as a consumption good is something people want to enjoy, rather than to use as a means of greater economic production" (Havighurst, 1967, p. 516). This means not only greater attention to the arts but also greater concern with education as it relates to living here and now.

One reason why the demands of black students are often easier to deal with in spite of the rhetoric is that they are directed in good part to the opportunity and production functions. These are understandable issues in our established ways of operating. Demands on the consumption side present new problems. For the blacks, however, there is sometimes the complexity of attempting to achieve all three objectives at the same time.

The case of educational institutions, moreover, is not unique. The interests and expectations of consumers of goods and services no longer remain disregarded either by industry or government. Outside pressures and demands are increasingly responded to with greather attention by most organizations, however inadequately or belatedly. In the health care field, for example, hospitals slowly are becoming more responsive to the health care expectations of an increasingly better educated and more demanding clientèle who now see comprehensive health care as a right. At the same time, as the costs of care continue to rise at staggering rates, the quest for quality care is accompanied by demands for public controls, higher organizational efficiency, and even reorganization of the entire health system (Bugbee, 1969; McNerney, 1969; Sibery, 1969; TIME, 1969; U.S. News and World Report, 1969). Hospitals are being pressured from all directions to innovate and experiment with new patterns of internal social organization and more effective forms of operation in the areas of administration, staffing, organizational rewards for members, community relations, and the utilization of both new health knowledge and new social-psychological knowledge (Georgopoulos, 1964, 1969). As a consequence, they are being forced to be not only more community-oriented but also more sensitive to the interests and contributions of their various groups of members at all levels (Georgopoulos & Matejko, 1967). More generally, partly as a result of affluence and economic growth, organizations in all areas are becoming more open systems and less immune to social forces in their environment.

Economic affluence and the decline in traditional authority are related to a shift in motive patterns in our society. Maslow (1943) developed the notion years ago of a hierarchy of motives ranging from biological needs, through security, love, and belongingness, to ego needs of self-esteem, self-development, and self-actualization. His thesis was that the motives at the bottom of the hierarchy were imperative in their demands and made the higher level motives relatively ineffectual. Once these lower level needs are assured satisfaction, however, the higher level needs take over and become all-important.

Maslow's thesis has abundant support among the young people in our educational system. They are less concerned with traditional economic careers than was once the case. A recent study reported only 14 per cent of the graduates of a leading university planning business careers, compared with 39 per cent five years earlier and 70 per cent in 1928 (Marrow, Bowers, & Seashore, 1967). Engineering schools similarly are experiencing falling enrollments.

Our society has been called, with considerable justification, the *achieving society* (McClelland, 1961). The content analysis of children's readers by de Charms and Moeller (1962) shows that a great rise in achievement themes occurred in the last part of the 19th century, but a great decline in this emphasis has occurred in recent decades.

The decline in the older motive patterns has one direct consequence for all organizations. Extrinsic rewards such as pay, job security, fringe benefits, and conditions of work are no longer so attractive. Younger people are demanding intrinsic job satisfactions as well. They are less likely to accept the notion of deferring gratifications in the interests of some distant career.

In most organizations today the dominant motives of members are the higher-order ego and social motives—particularly those for personal gratification, independence, self-expression, power, and self-actualization (Argyris, 1964; Blake & Mouton, 1968; Georgopoulos, 1970; Georgopoulos & Matejko, 1967; Herzberg, 1968; Likert, 1967; Marrow, Bowers, & Seashore, 1967; McGregor, 1960; Schein, 1965). Increasingly, expressive needs and the pursuit of immediate and intrinsic rewards are outstripping economic achievement motives in importance, both in the work situation and outside. Correspondingly, the dominant incentives and rewards required for member compliance, role performance, and organizational effectiveness are social and psychological rather than economic (Blake & Mouton, 1968; Etzioni, 1964; Georgopoulos, 1970; Georgopoulos & Matejko, 1967; Herzberg, 1968; Likert, 1967; Marrow, Bowers, & Seashore, 1967; McGregor, 1960). Even at the rank-and-file level, where economic motives are especially strong, there is now more concern on the part of unions for other than bread-and-butter issues, and contract negotiations often stall on matters of policy, control, and work rules rather than money. As a result of these shifts, there is pressure for a place in the decision-making structure of the system from all groups and members in organizations, and there is a growing need for meaningful participation in the affairs of the organization by all concerned at all levels.

The forms which newly aroused ego motives take can vary, but at present there are a number of patterns familiar to all of us. First there is the emphasis upon self-determination or self-expression, or "doing one's thing." Second is the demand for self-development and self-actualization, making the most of one's own talents and abilities. Third is the unleashing of power drives. The hippies represent the first emphasis of self-expression, some of the leftist leaders the emphasis upon power. Fourth is the outcome of the other three, a blanket rejection of established values—a revolutionary attack upon the existing system as exploitative and repressive of the needs of individuals.

With the need for self-expression goes the ideology of the importance of spontaneity; of the wholeness of human experience; the reliance upon emotions; and the attack upon the fragmentation, the depersonalization, and the restrictions of the present social forms. It contributes to the anti-intellectualism of the student movement and is reminiscent of the romanticism of an older period in which Wordsworth spoke of the intellect as that false secondary power which multiplies delusions. Rationality is regarded as rationalization.

Not only are we witnessing significant shifts in the economic and value patterns of society but they are happening at a very fast rate. Probably there has always been some conflict between the older and younger generations, but in the past there has been more time to socialize children into older patterns and the patterns were of longer duration, thus preventing serious lags and social dislocation. History is becoming less relevant for predicting change. It is difficult to know what the generation now entering high school will be like when they enter college.

All organizations face a period of trouble and turmoil because of these changes, which affect all three levels of integration in social systems. Some of the basic values of the social system are under fire, such as representative democracy of the traditional, complex type, the belief in private property, conventional morality, the importance of work and of economic achievement, the good life as the conventional enjoyment of the products of mass culture. The Protestant Ethic (Weber, 1958) is no longer pervasive and paramount in our society.

The norms legitimized by societal values of orderly procedures and of conformity to existing rules until they are changed by socially sanctioned procedures are also brought into question. The rebels emphasize not law and order but justice, and justice as they happen to see it. It is interesting that President Nixon, the spokesman for the Establishment, modified his plea for law and order by stressing law, order, and justice. The challenge to the norms of any system is especially serious, since it is genuinely revolutionary or anarchistic in implication, whether voiced by official revolutionaries or reformers. If the legitimate channels for change are abandoned and the resort is to direct action, then people are going outside the system. If enough do, the system collapses.

At the level of role integration there is also real difficulty. As has already been noted, extrinsic rewards have lost some of their importance in our affluent society. Moreover, the usual set of roles in an organization segmentalize individuals, and our ever-advancing technology adds to the problem. A role is only partially inclusive of personality at most levels of the organization. This fractionation runs counter to the needs for wholeness and for self-expression. Increasing specialization everywhere exacerbates the problem (Etzioni, 1964; Georgopoulos, 1966; Georgopoulos, 1970; Georgopoulos & Mann, 1962; Likert, 1967; J. D. Thompson, 1967; V. Thompson 1961). It engenders coordination and integration difficulties for organizations and their members because it results in greater organizational complexity and more intensive interdependence among unlike participants who must relate to one another and to the system and whose efforts must be collectively regulated (Georgopoulos, 1966; Georgopoulos & Mann, 1962; Morton, 1964; V. Thompson, 1961; Wieland, 1965). Role specialization is the main social invention available with which man can cope with the problems of the explosion of knowledge in our times, for specialization makes possible both the utilization of available knowledge and the development of new knowledge. But, at the same time, specialization leads to fractionation and diversity that make the integration of members into the system all the more difficult to attain.

In linking the changed patterns of many of the younger generation to societal changes, we want to emphasize that it is an error to simplify the problem as a younger-older generation conflict. It is broader and deeper than that, and many of the developing trends predate the present student generation. In fact, the revolt started with people now in their sixties, if not earlier. *We* were the ones to attack the inequities of bureaucratic society, the ones to raise children in democratic practices and to think for themselves. The older generations furnished the ideology of the present student movements. Try to find any ideology in these movements which is not a bastardized version of old revolutionary and romantic doctrines. *We* started the rebellion and now we are astonished to find that we are the "establishment."

This is one reason why organizations have been so vulnerable to atttack. Older citizens do not rally to their support because they feel that the rebels are in good part right. Or else why should we so often hear it stated, "We agree with your objectives but we don't like your tactics"? Nathan Glazer (1969) has shown, however, that this vague sentiment is based upon a failure to come to grips with the significant issues.

The dynamic nature of our society makes imperative greater attention to processes of adaptation. In the past, industrial organizations, because of their dependence upon a market, have developed adaptive subsystems of planning, research, and development. The major emphasis has been, however, upon production inputs, upon product development, upon finding new markets and exploiting old ones, upon technology in improving their productive system. Only minor attention has been placed upon social inputs or upon restructuring the organization to meet the psychological needs of members. Technological innovation without social innovation has been the rule, and exclusive concern with technical and economic efficiency has undermined the social and psychological efficiency of the system to the detriment of organizational effectiveness and adaptability.

Traditionally, organizations have shown much more concern for the technology of work than for their social inputs and human assets. They have been more concern with providing a safe and attractive physical work environment than with creating and maintaining an equally attractive social and psychological work climate for the members. With the emphasis for technical and economic efficiency, they have paid much more attention to recruiting and selecting members with the "proper" training and aptitude for filling inflexibly defined jobs than to problems of member attitudes, needs, and values. The approach has been to fit the man to the job rather than the other way around, and organizational role redefinition has been largely disregarded as a problem-solving mechanism. Organizational restructuring to improve the adaptability of the system has been abhorred and resisted. Most organizations have avoided social innovation and renovation and have sought technological innovation as the answer to all of their problems. Correspondingly, in relating to their members, they have been concerned with authority-based, superior-subordinate relations more than with social relations, relying more on economic incentives and rewards and less on social-psychological motivation and compensation.

Because of the changes in society just discussed, however, the situation is now changing within organizations as well. The conditions for effective role performance, job satisfaction, member integration into the system, and organizational effectiveness and adaptability demand different organization-member relations than in the past. For organizations to survive and perform their functions effectively in the future, some sizable proportion of their resources will have to be committed to enlarging their adaptive subsystems to deal more adequately with external relations and new social inputs. Social effectiveness will have to be added to productive efficiency as an important objective.

Better adaptive subsystems are now needed not only in industrial organizations but in all complex organizations, including educational and health institutions. The case of hospitals is instructive. Continuous progress in medicine, nursing, and allied health professions and occupations, advances in medical technology, the professionalization of hospital administration, and the explosion of knowledge witnessed inside and outside the health field have made a strong impact upon the traditional social organization of the hospital system. The result is a gradual redefinition of the institutional role of the hospital as the health center in the total framework of health-related institutions. Such redefinition, however, is being forced by public expectations and demands from without and pressures from nonmedical members in the prevailing power structure, rather than from planned social innovation within the system (Georgopoulos, 1969; Georgopoulos, 1970; Georgopoulos & Matejko, 1967). Redefinition is taking place and must be accomplished along with proper internal organizational restructuring, however, in the context of current health trends and societal health conceptions—for example, the Medicare program, the recent development of regional medical programs, the growing emphasis on comprehensive health planning, the promulgated national goal of adequate health care for all, and the widespread concern for improvements in care coverage, quality, and cost.

These recent changes in the health field, along with the major changes in society discussed earlier, have strong and concrete implications for the kind of organizational restructuring that is feasible and appropriate for the hospital as a complex, sociotechnical, problem-solving system. Today's hospital is still ruled by three dominant decision-making centers—trustees, physicians, and administrators (Georgopoulos & Mann, 1962; Georgopoulos & Matejko, 1967). The above trends argue, however, for better recognition of the contributions of nurses and nonmedical groups and for a broader base of decision making. They argue for an interaction-influence structure which transcends the conventional tripartite arrangement and which can truly encompass all participants regardless of their professional affiliation or hierarchical position in the system. The traditional maintenance mechanisms and adaptive structures of the organization (formal authority, rule enforcement, medical dominance, identification with the system primarily on the basis of moral values and service motives, influence and rewards according to professional status and hierarchical position) which have been successful in the past are clearly becoming less and less effective (Georgopoulos, 1969; Georgopoulos & Matejko, 1967). Inside and outside the system the premises of the traditional structure no longer remain unchallenged, and new bases for organizational adaptation are therefore required.

Similar problems, evident in all large-scale organizations, await solution. Without an adequate adaptive subsystem to modify and filter new inputs leading to planned change, two things can happen: The new potential inputs can be summarily rejected; the organizational structure becomes rigid and the problems are postponed and often intensified. Or the inputs slip into the system and are incorporated in undigested fashion; there is erosion of basic values and the system loses its identity. It does not acquire a formal death certificate but for practical purposes it has been replaced. If a university were to accept research inputs uncritically from the Defense Department, for example, it could end up as a branch of the military and not as an institution for advancing science. Sometimes it happens that in organizations the first response of blanket rejection and rigidity cannot be maintained over time and the opposite reaction of wholesale acceptance of any and all demands follows. For example, a university may show rigidity to suggested reforms at first, and then, as pressure mounts, capitulate completely without critical evaluation of the suggested changes. To complicate matters, both rigidity and uncritical incorporation can occur in different parts of the same organization.

References

Argyris, C. *Integrating the individual and the organization.* New York: Wiley, 1964.

Berkowitz, L., & Daniels, Louise R. Responsibility and dependency. *J. abnorm. soc. Psychol., 1963, 66,* 429-437.

Blake, R. R., & Mouton, Jane S. *Corporate excellence through grid organization development.* Houston, Tex.: Gulf, 1968.

Blau, P. M. Justice in social exchange. *Sociolog. Inquiry,* 1964, *24,* 199-200.

Bugbee, G. Delivery of health care services: Long range outlook. The Univer. of Michigan *Medical Center J.,* 1969, *35,* 75-76.

Dalton, M. Conflicts between staff and line managerial officers. *Amer. sociolog. Rev.,* 1950, *15,* 342-351.

de Charms, R., & Moeller, G. H. Values expressed in children's readers. *J. abnorm. soc. Psychol.,* 1962, *64,* 136-142.

Etzioni, A. *Modern organizations.* Englewood Cliffs, N.J.: Prentice-Hall, 1964.

Georgopoulos, B. S. Hospital organization and administration. *Hospital Admin.,* 1964, *9,* 23-35.

Georgopoulos, B. S. The hospital system and nursing: Some basic problems and issues. *Nursing Forum,* 1966, *5,* 8-35.

Georgopoulos, B. S. The general hospital as an organization: A social-psychological viewpoint. The Univer. of Michigan *Medical Center J.,* 1969, *35,* 94-97.

Georgopoulos, B. S. An open-system theory model for organizational research: The case of the contemporary general hospital. In A. R. Negandhi and J. P. Schwitter (Eds.), *Organizational behavior models.* Kent, Ohio: Kent State Univer., 1970. Pp. 33-70.

Georgopoulos, B. S., & Mann, F. C. *The community general hospital.* New York: Macmillan, 1962.

Georgopoulos, B. S., & Matejko, A. The American general hospital as a complete social system. *Health Services Res.,* 1967, *2,* 76-112.

Georgopoulos, B. S., & Wieland, G. F. *Nationwide study of coordination and patient care in voluntary hospitals,* No. 2187. Ann Arbor, Mich.: Institute for Social Research, The Univer. of Michigan, 1964.

Glazer, N. The campus crucible 1. Student politics and the university. *Atlantic Monthly,* July 1969, *224,* 43-53.

Golomb, N. Managing without sanctions or rewards. *Mgmt of Personnel Q.*, 1968, *7*, 22-28.

Gouldner, A. W. The norm of reciprocity: A preliminary statement. *Amer. sociolog, Rev.*, 1960, *25*, 161-178.

Havighurst, R. J. The social and educational implications of interinstitutional cooperation in higher education. In L. C. Howard (Ed.), *Interinstitutional cooperation in higher education*. Milwaukee: Univer. of Wisconsin, 1967. Pp. 508-523.

Herzberg, F. One more time: How do you motivate employees? *Harvard bus. Rev.*, 1968, *46*, 53-62.

Katz, D., & Kahn, R. L. *The social psychology of organizations*. New York: Wiley, 1966.

Likert, R. *The human organization: Its management and value*. New York: McGraw-Hill, 1967.

Marrow, A. J. Bowers, D. G., & Seashore, S. E. *Management by participation*. New York: Harper and Row, 1967.

Maslow, A. H. A theory of human motivation. *Psycholog. Rev.*, 1943, *50*, 370-396.

McClelland, D. *The achieving society*. New York: D. Van Nostrand, 1961.

McGregor, D. M. *The human side of enterprise*. New York: McGraw-Hill, 1960.

McNerney, W. J. Does America need a new health system? The Univer. of Michigan *Medical Center J.*, 1969, *35*, 82-87.

Morton, J. A. From research to technology. *Int. Sci. & Technol.*, May 1964, Issue No. 29, 82-92.

Parsons, T. *Structure and process in modern society*. Glencoe, Ill.: Free Press, 1960.

Presthus, R. *The organization*. London: Tavistock Publications, 1958.

Schein, E. H. *Organizational psychology*. Englewood Cliffs, N.J.: Prentice-Hall, 1965.

Sibery, D. E. Our social responsibilities as health professionals and university center hospitals. The Univer. of Michigan *Medical Center J.*, 1969, *35*, 8-93.

Thompson, J. D. *Organizations in action*. New York: McGraw-Hill, 1967.

Thompson, V. *Modern organization*. New York: Knopf, 1961.

TIME Magazine, Medicine—the plight of the U.S. patient. February 21, 1969, *93*, 53-58.

Trist, E. L., Higgin, G. W., Murray, H., & Pollock, A. B. *Organizational choice*. London: Tavistock Publications, 1963.

U.S. News & World Report. How to improve medical care. March 24, 1969, *66*, 41-46.

Weber, M. *The theory of social and economic organization* (A. M. Henderson & T. Parsons transl.). New York: Oxford Univer. Press, 1947.

Weber, M. *The protestant ethic and the rise of capitalism* (T. Parsons transl.). New York: Scribner, 1958.

Wieland, G. F. Complexity and coordination in organizations. Unpublished doctoral dissertation, The Univer. of Michigan, 1965.

8

Institutionalization of the Aged: Effects on Behavior

MORTON A. LIEBERMAN

The effects of institutionalization on the psychological well-being and physical integrity of aged adults has been a question of humanitarian interest since the late nineteenth century and of scientific inquiry for 30 years. This paper assesses current knowledge and research strategies regarding the effects of institutional living on the elderly and delineates the contributions future research might make to policy formation.

For the purpose of this review, institutions are defined as residential facilities providing one or more central services that meet some particular need of the client and/or society. Studies of geriatric centers, nursing homes, domiciliaries, and chronic disease units are included, as well as facilities that serve a large number of aged but are not exclusively oriented toward them, such as mental hospitals. Such settings imply permanent or indefinite residence involving a major change from a community living pattern. Temporary institutionalization (such as brief hospitalizations) or settings which do not provide multiple centralized services (such as retirement villages) are not included. Empirical studies on the institutionalization of children and of psychiatric patients are discussed to illustrate gaps in knowledge regarding the aged.

FROM: *Journal of Gerontology*, Vol. 24, July 1969, pp. 330-340.

EFFECTS OF INSTITUTIONALIZATION

It is commonly believed that most institutions have deleterious effects caused by the "dehumanizing" and "depersonalizing" characteristics of institutional environments. Townsend (1962) succinctly summarizes this general view.

> In the institution people live communally with a minimum of privacy and yet their relationships with each other are slender. Many subsist in a kind of defensive shell of isolation. Their mobility is restricted, and they have little access to a general society. The social experiences are limited, and the staff lead a rather separate existence from them. They are subtly oriented toward a system in which they submit to orderly routine, non-creative occupation, and cannot exercise as much self-determination. They are deprived of intimate family relationships and can rarely find substitutes which seem to be more than a pale imitation of those enjoyed by most people in a general community. The result for the individual seems fairly often to be a gradual process of depersonalization. He has too little opportunity to develop the talents he possesses and they atrophy through disuse. He may become resigned and depressed and may display no interest in the future or in things not immediately personal. He sometimes becomes apathetic, talks little, and lacks initiative. His personal habits and toilet may deteriorate. Occasionally he seems to withdraw into a private world of fantasy.

Such a view has been associated with the contention that institutions for the aged are often "dumping grounds," housing many who need not live there. This view is countered by Shanas (1961) and others who suggest, on the basis of survey data, that the majority of institutionalized aged have real needs they are attempting to solve via the institution. Whether alternatives exist to meet these needs is unknown, and whether, in fact, alternatives are needed depends at least in part on whether institutionalization really does have deleterious effects and, if so, to what extent and in what ways.

The common sense view that institutions have deleterious effects on the psychological well-being and physical survival of aged adults appears to be supported by a host of empirical studies.

A representative compilation of studies of the elderly residing in homes for the aged, domiciliaries, and nursing homes suggests that they share the following characteristics: poor adjustment, depression and unhappiness, intellectual ineffectiveness because of increased rigidity and low energy (but not necessarily intellectual incompetence), negative self-image, feelings of personal insignificance and impotency, and a view of self as old. Residents tend to be docile, submissive, show a low range of interests and activities, and to live in the past rather than the future. They are withdrawn and unresponsive in relationship to others. There is some suggestion that they have increased anxiety, which at times focuses on feelings of death (Ames, 1954; Chalfen, 1956; Coe, 1967; Davidson & Kurglov, 1952; Dorken, 1951; Eicker, 1959; Fink, 1957; Fox, 1950; Lakin, 1960; Laverty, 1950; Lepkowsky, 1954; Lieberman & Lakin, 1963; Mason, 1954; Pan, 1950; Pollack, Karp, & Goldfarb, 1962; Shrut, 1958; Swenson, 1961; Tuckman & Lorge, 1952). Other investigators (Camargo & Preston, 1945; Kay, Norris, & Post, 1956; Lieberman, 1961; Roth, 1955; Whittier & Williams, 1956) have reported marked increases in mortality rates for aged persons entering mental institutions or homes for the aged.

These studies clearly demonstrate that aged persons residing in a variety of institutional settings are psychologically worse off and likely to die sooner than aged persons living in the community. Without additional information all of this research is worthless, however, in determining whether life in the institution induces such effects. Difference between institutional and community residents does not of itself mean that institutionalization is the essential variable that created the differences. Before such a conclusion can be entertained, aged persons in institutions and aged persons living in the community must be shown comparable, differing only in respect to where they live. It must also be shown that the characteristics of institutional life, *per se*, and not other factors associated with becoming institutionalized, induce these deleterious effects.

SELECTION BIASES

How many of the effects attributed to living in institutions can be explained on the basis of population differences between those living in the community and those residing in institutions? Such an approach might explain the negative psychological characteristics of institutionalized aged as a product of disease (physical or mental), or as a product of personality characteristics associated with resolving crises of old age by seeking institutional settings, or as a product of certain life crises that brought about institutionalization. Three types of evidence are relevant to this issue: (*a*) population survey data, (*b*) longitudinal or follow-up studies of institutionalized aged, and (*c*) studies that attempt to identify the particular populations from which specific institutions draw their residents.

Population surveys.—Since the turn of the century the proportion of aged residing in institutions has steadily increased. This trend, coupled with increased longevity, has meant that institutions have been used more and more to cope with major incapacitating physical or mental illness. It would be reasonable to conclude, therefore, that aged residing in institutions are physically and mentally different from community aged.

Studies of particular samples of institutionalized aged, however, in contrast to simple population statistics, show that significant proportions of the elderly residing in institutions do not differ physically or mentally from their community counterparts. Gitlitz (1956), utilizing morbidity, mortality, and psychiatric disorder statistics from a large home for the aged, suggests that the incidence of specific types of morbidity may not differ from the community aged. These apparent discrepancies between population statistics and studies carried out on particular small samples stem to some extent from the under-estimation of psychiatric and physical morbidity in community samples and the relative over-estimation in the institutional samples because of better diagnostic techniques.

The occurrence of physical illness among the institutionalized aged takes on added significance because of the suggestive evidence (Birren, 1959; Coe, 1962) that physical illness, even at preclinical levels, affects psychological status. If it could be shown that logical characteristics attributed to institutionalization were significantly related to physical illness, the evidence for selective factors would be appreciably strengthened. To date there is no strong empirical evidence demonstrating this relationship.

It has also been shown (Goldfarb, 1962) that in particular types of institutions such as homes for the aged, the incidence of chronic brain syndrome varies, ranging from rates of one per cent or less to rates that parallel those found in state mental hospitals. Such variations, even among a limited group of institutions for the aged, lend further weight to the probability that some of the effects attributed to living in an institution may be associated with other than institutional factors.

Longitudinal studies.—As yet, few longitudinal studies of the aged exist which include data about the period before actual residence in the institution. One study, however, (Lieberman, Prock, & Tobin, 1968) revealed considerably less psychological deterioration when institutionalized aged were measured relative to their own pre-institutional characteristics than cross-sectional comparisons of institutional to non-institutional populations would suggest. This adds to the evidence that some of the effects attributed to institutional environments might more appropriately be accounted for by selection.

Studies on selection.—Who come to institutions and why they come is an exceedingly complex issue that no single study answers. There are several studies that are directly applicable. Unfortunately most (Bortner, 1962; Fogel, Swepston, Zintek, Vernier, Fitzgerald, Marnocha, & Weschler, 1956; Webb, 1959) represent highly specialized populations among the institutionalized aged (VA domiciliaries). Although utilizing different methods, these investigators attribute psychological differences between institutionalized and community aged to selection processes. For example, Webb (1959) found that the type of individual who applies and resides in such institutions differs in specific socio-economic factors as well as personality variables—rigidity, stereotyped thinking, apathy, resignation, ego-eccentricity, passivity, strong needs for love, affection, and care. Many of these factors identifying the persons who apply are the same characteristics as those of "institutionalized populations." Lowenthal (1964), investigating pathways to mental institutions among the aged, found a particular type of interpersonal relationship differentiating those who enter from those who do not enter such institutions. These studies, although few in number and covering a limited range of institutions, point to an association between entering an institution and certain psychological or social characteristics. In contrast, a study comparing community residents, applicants for old age homes, and long-term residents of such homes (Lieberman, Prock, & Tobin, 1968) did not show personality characteristics or occurrences of crises events distinguishing those who entered institutions from those who remained in the community.

Population survey data can at best be suggestive; it cannot offer positive evidence that selection plays a role. Other studies, focused more directly on the selection issue, are limited in number and scope. There are, however, sufficient data to indicate that the differences between institutionalized and non-institutionalized aged are significantly influenced by the factor of selection. Institutionalized aged share some characteristics because of *who* they are and not *where* they are. On the other hand, the evidence for selection is not sufficient to explain all of the noxious effects associated with living in an institution.

ENVIRONMENTAL CHANGE

A number of investigators have studied the effects of radical environmental changes on the psychological well-being and physical survival of the aged. Many of these studies have involved changes from community living to life in an institution; others have studied relocation from one institutional setting to another. Some have investigated environmental changes that involve movement from one community setting to another. These studies are particularly relevant to the consideration of the effects of living in institutional settings. They suggest that the conditions associated with *moving* into an institution create many of the effects attributed to *living* in an institutional setting. The majority of these studies (Aldrich & Mendkoff, 1963; Blenkner, 1967; Goldfarb, Shahinian, & Turner, 1966; Jasnau, 1967; Lieberman, 1961) showed that changing the environment of elderly persons sharply increased the death rate.

While the studies of Lawton and Yaffe (1967) and Miller and Lieberman (1965) failed to show increased mortality, other negative effects were observed. In Lawton and Yaffe's study, the relocated group was judged to have declined more frequently on measures of health compared to the control group; in the Miller and Lieberman study, half the Ss declined either psychologically (occurrences of confusion, memory defects, bizarre behavior) or physically (hospitalization, restrictions of activity, health failures). A recent study (Lieberman et al., 1968) showed that many of the effects (on self-image, interpersonal relationships, mood-tone, etc.) ascribed to living in an institution were set in motion by the *decision to enter* an institution and occurred with maximum intensity prior to actual entrance. Fried (1963), in studying relocation forced by urban renewal, noted that many persons suffered serious depressive reactions subsequent to such relocation. He explained these effects in terms of a fragmentation of spatial and group identity. Friedsam (1961), who studied reactions to disaster, showed that events which markedly changed living patterns created profound psychological distress and were particularly destructive for the aged.

Although, over-all, the evidence suggests that radical environmental change for the aged leads to destructive physical processes and has noxious psychological effects, some investigators present data which suggest that more precision is required in understanding which conditions and what types of aged will experience such environmental changes as severe crises.

Dobson and Patterson (1961), Epstein and Simon (1967), and Stotsky (1967) studied elderly mentally ill moved for "therapeutic" purposes to nursing homes, boarding homes, or homes for the aged. Here, relocation (many of the Ss had lived in institutions most of their adult lives) did not produce massive death rates or increased psychological or physical disabilities. Carp's study (1967) of elderly persons moving into apartment dwellings showed an increase in satisfaction and adjustment. Goldfarb et al. (1966) and Donahue (1965) have suggested that under certain conditions (which are at this juncture mostly unknown) some individuals entering or being relocated from one institution to another experienced positive (ego-enhancing) effects.

This pattern of negative and positive findings suggests a number of potentially fruitful hypotheses that are beginning to gain investigative attention. Such studies can add significantly to knowledge about the noxious effects associated with institutionalization and, more important, to specifying the conditions associated with negative effects.

Data are also beginning to accumulate about the characteristics of people who are vulnerable to environmental change. A number of investigators have found that psychiatric disturbance and cognitive malfunctioning (Aldrich & Mendkoff, 1963; Goldfarb, 1966) are positively associated with risk. Studies investigating personality patterns, depression, etc., have also suggested associations with risk (Aldrich & Mendkoff, 1963; Miller & Lieberman, 1965). Goldfarb et al. (1966) have suggested that cognitive intactness is associated with improvement under relocation.

Evidence concerning the conditions which affect reactions to change is only beginning to appear in the literature, and the multiplicity of theoretical propositions and technical problems makes the findings presently rather tentative. Voluntary or involuntary change (Lawton & Yaffe, 1967) and the adequacy of preparation[1] are associated with vulnerability to change. Jasnau (1967) suggests that "massed" relocations without adequate "warning" are destructive. The meaning of institutionalization for the individual may affect his reactions. The attitudes of the elderly toward institutional arrangements closely parallel the common societal stereotypes about such institutions. Kleemeier (1960) suggested that older persons exhibit a generalized negative feeling toward all special settings for the aged. Montgomery (1965), studying rural aged, found a consistent desire to remain in the present residence and equated this with highly-valued independence. Shanas (1961) found aged adults associated moving with loss of independence, prelude to death, rejection by the children. Lieberman and Lakin (1963) found aged awaiting institutionalization attached symbols of fear, rejection, and dread to the event. Tobin (1968) found thema of extreme loss in a group facing institutionalization.

Although data are not available which bear directly on the relationships of such feelings of loss to subsequent effects of institutionalization, studies in other areas on the effects of loss are highly suggestive (Yarrow, Blank, Quinn, Youmans, and Stein, 1963). Research on the sequelae of widowhood has shown some of the same patterns as for institutionalization: increased mortality, incidence of physical disorder, withdrawal, and depression. A number of investigators have associated psychological loss with the onset of physical illness. Research on childhood hospitalization supports the view that the feeling of loss is a major contributor to the upsetting aspects of institutionalization. Inquiry based on the psychology of loss may offer a more effective framework for identifying factors leading to noxious effects of institutionalization than analyses of institutional characteristics. Unfortunately, the state of current reseasrch on the psychology of loss makes it impossible to determine if all losses are psychologically equivalent. The degree of specificity such a model would offer is unknown, e.g., whether loss associated with widowhood is analogous in detail to loss surrounding institutionalization.

Characteristics of environmental change have also been studied in terms of "overload." To what extent change is disruptive and destructive depends upon the relationship between the characteristics of the two

---

[1]Only anecdotal data are available for the aged. Good empirical data can be found in studies of the hospitalization of children (Prugh, Staub, Sands, Kirschbaum, & Lenihan, 1953; Vaughan, 1967) which show mitigation of the deleterious effects of hospitalization.

environments, a question that is currently being investigated. The larger the difference between old and new situations, the greater the possibility that the aged individual will need to develop adaptive responses often beyond his capacity. In this light, the effect of an institution can be viewed less as a product of its quality or characteristics than of the degree to which it forces the person to make new adaptive responses or employ adaptive responses from the previous environment. It is possible that some of the current trends aimed at "de-institutionalizing" institutions, e.g., making them more open to the outside community, less congregant, etc., are effective because they permit the use of prior adaptive responses.

This review of the effects of selection and degree of environmental change suggests that these two factors may explain many of the deleterious effects on aged which are associated with living in an institution.

INSTITUTIONAL EFFECTS—STUDIES OF INSTITUTIONAL SAMPLES

Another group of studies which bear on the effects of institutionalization are not subject to selection biases created by comparing institutional to non-institutional populations or to the unkown effects of radical environmental change itself. These studies have used one of three design strategies: study of the psychological well-being of institutional persons as a function of alterations made in the structure of the institution; study of the effects on behavior of the length of time spent in an institution; and comparison of the effects on individuals of residence in various institutional settings. Although these strategies minimize some methodological pitfalls inherent in the previously discussed studies, they raise some new problems.

ALTERATION IN INSTITUTIONAL STRUCTURE

The view that certain characteristics of institutionalized persons (which were previously thought part of a disease process, such as the withdrawal and apathetic behavior of schizophrenics) were associated with life in an institution has in large measure been supported by evidence from studies of institutional change. A large body of descriptive anecdotal material and some controlled studies in mental hospitals beginning with the classic descriptions of Stanton and Schwartz (1954), suggest that hospital structure has an impact upon the inmates and that certain changes in such structures may be ameliorative. Much of this change has been directed toward therapeutic goals, e.g., the change from custodial to therapeutic care in mental hospitals. Although studies specific to the aged are less frequent, the findings agree with the broad findings in the field—that certain types of alteration in the social-physical world have ameliorative effects and that such changes are toward "de-institutionalizing" the institution (Greenblatt, York, & Brown, 1955).

Some current works (Gottesman, 1963; Kahana, 1968) are illustrative. Kahana experimented with age-segregated and age non-segregated environments and found that the non-segregated environment led to an increase in social interaction and emotional responsivity and toward improvement in mental functioning. Her samples were composed mainly of new admissions, thus making the results for the purpose of this review only suggestive. Gottesman's study also suggested that alterations in the physical or social structure of institutions for aged mental patients can mitigate negative behavior.

Despite such results that indicate a positive association between environmental qualities and psychological functioning, a research strategy based only on alterations in the environment cannot make the critical contribution to the central questions on delimiting the general psychological effects of living in an institutional environment. The characteristics of the institutionalized mental patient — apathy, withdrawal, etc. — may be a product of the disease which is ameliorated or changed by alterations in the environment. However, changes in behavior do not demonstrate that a *particular* institutional environment was directly associated with those maladaptive behaviors. Moreover, the generaly positive results produced by most therapeutic millieu programs in hospitals for the mentally ill strongly suggest the possibility of a "Hawthorne" effect. These considerations, in addition to the pragmatic problems of making salient alterations in many institutional structures, suggest that this research strategy has limited usefulness in determining whether in general an institution for the elderly has noxious effects and which of its characteristics can be associated with such effects.

LENGTH OF INSTITUTIONALIZATION

Several investigators have attempted to isolate the effects of living in an institution by measuring behavior of Ss who live in a particular institution for varying amounts of time. Although potentially offering a reasonable method for specifying the noxious effects of institutional living, the yield from this method has been limited. Townsend (1962) found that those residing less than a year in an institution did not differ from residents of 10 years or more. Webb (1959), on the other hand, suggested that those who had lived in institutions for long periods of time indicated more concern about re-entry into the community and less willingness to attempt it.

Ongoing work (Lieberman, Tobin, & Slover, 1969) suggests a relationship between emotional responsivity and length of residence in institutions; however, most analyses reported in the literature have yielded few positive associations between length of time and psychological effects. As is all too often, a characteristic of research in the general area of institutional effects, "negative" results are often noncontributory. The methodological errors make such results too ambiguous for use. For example, the lack of significant findings may be associated with difficulties in method; length of time in an institution is associated with a biased population (discharge or death) and some investigators have not taken this factor into account. Given the relatively homogeneous populations in institutions, the need for sensitive measurement is increased, and most studies have reported results based upon crude data that may not discriminate existing difference.

COMPARATIVE ANALYSIS

Studies comparing a variety of institutions offer the best potential for isolating specific effects on the psychological behavior of the aged and for determining the environmental characteristics associated with these effects. Overall, the promise of this approach has not as yet been fulfilled. Townsend (1962) compared various types of institutions in a sample of 173 institutions. Utilizing scales based on adequacy ratings of physical facilities, staffing and services, mobility, freedom in daily life and social provisions, he suggested that differences in occupations, the number of visitors received, and the amount of mobility occurred between "good" and "bad" institutions. Townsend's evidence unfortunately did not provide information associating the quality of institutions and psychological characteristics attributed to institutional living, nor is it possible to determine from this study how much these institutions differed in populations served.

Dobson and Patterson (1961) compared geriatric mental patients living in nursing homes to patients living in state mental hospitals. Their analysis of behavioral ratings suggested no difference between the two groups. In a similar study, Epstein and Simon (1967) compared nursing homes and state hospital patients and found results comparable to those of Dobson and Patterson.

Coe (1962), using a model for assessing institutional structure, found some association between the degree of depersonalization of environment and the effects on self-imagery. Bennett, Nahemow, and Zubin (1964), suggested that the more total the institution (based on such items as orientation of activities, scheduling of activities, provisions for dissemination of rules and standards of conduct, provisions for allocation of staff time and observation of the behavior of inmates, types of sanction system, how personal property is dealt with, decision-making about the use of private property, pattern of recruitment, voluntary-involuntary and residential pattern, congregate versus private) the greater its depersonalizing effects. Schrut (1958) compared 60 Ss, 30 living in "apartment-like" dwellings associated with old age homes and 30 living in the more central "institutional" home, found that the Ss living in the apartments (more like their previous living arrangements) showed less anxiety about their health and less fear or preoccupation with death that Ss living in the central facility.

The studies in this area that have produced positive findings (an association between institutional characteristics and effects on persons living in those institutions) have had two common characteristics: (a) the different institutions were compared using a conceptual framework for measuring differences among institutions rather than making comparisons based upon types of institutions, and (b) the effects on the psychological well-being of the residents were measured by instruments that were apparently more sensitive than the more commonly used rating scale approach.

None of the studies surveyed has met the problem of differences in population found among different institutions of a similar type (for example, Goldfarb's (1962) report of extreme ranges in cognitive impairment among homes for the aged.) Thus, it is unknown how many of the positive findings can be attributed to population differences. To make the method of comparative analysis effective, the population characteristics of institutions must be taken into account, perhaps by the use of multivariate statistical procedure (use of complex statistical methods is rare in research on institutionalization).

An overview of the findings available to date suggests the tentative conclusion that despite the appearance of what seem to be "good" and "bad" institutions, those characteristics that are instrumental in influencing the behavior of the individuals residing in them are shared by all institutions, and these common characteristics may be more salient in producing negative influences than those characteristics that differentiate one institution from another. An instructive parallel can be found in the studies of the effects of interpersonal aspects that differentiate institutions catering to children. Such studies (Vernon, Foley, Sipowicz & Schulman, 1965) have by and large failed to show clearcut relationships between the degree and kind of maladaptive reactions of children and the particular characteristics of various institutions.

SUMMARY AND RECOMMENDATIONS
FOR FUTURE RESEARCH

The common stereotype about the destructive influences on the aged of living in institutional settings is overdrawn. Many of the supposed psychological effects are characteristics of the person *prior* to his coming to an institution (and are related in part to the reasons for institutionalization) and some appear to be associated with aspects of *entering* the institution (making a radical change in the environment) which occurred before the individual actually entered the institution. The only long-term effect of living in an institution that can be demonstrated is the increasing difficulty of re-entering the community and making appropriate adaptations. There appear to be considerably more destructive effects associated with radical environmental change (*entrance* into institutions) than with residence in an institution.

These conclusions must be viewed as highly tentative, however, because methodological biases in this area of inquiry are severe.

MEASUREMENT OF EFFECTS

1. The number of procedures used to assess institutional effects is as large as the number of studies. The use of some of these instruments is open to serious question (for example, the Rorschach) because of "set" problems with aged populations. Moreover, generalization across studies of institutional effects has been restricted because different instruments have been used to measure the same variable. In studying rigidity, for example, Davidson and Kruglov (1952) used the Rorschach, whereas Eicker (1959) used the Schaie test. Studies of rigidity have suggested that it is a construct highly dependent upon particular tests.

A common core of measures to be used by investigators is suggested. This is not contingent upon development of new methods but only upon more concern for comparability in the use of those currently existent. (The recent history of psychotherapy research is instructive on this point. The increasing comparability of measures, even without increasing theoretical or methodological sophistication, has added appreciably to the findings in a field that not too long ago resembled the present state of research on institutions.)

2. Studies in this area have tended to show negative effects in proportion to the sensitivity of their measures. Studies in this area have tended to show negative effects in proportion to the sensitivity of their measures. Studies that have relied on general behavioral description, rating scales, etc., have tended to show fewer negative characteristics associated with

institutionalization than studies that have relied on highly discriminating, more direct (usually test) measures. (This observation parallels those made of studies of the effects of maternal deprivation in childhood [Ainsworth, 1966].) The use of refined instrumentation is suggested.

3. By and large, measures have been oriented toward negative effects. Obviously, some aged persons may improve in an institution. The measures used and the methods of analysis may thus have overlooked certain ameliorative characteristics of institutionalization. (Results in psychotherapy outcome studies, uniformly oriented toward determining improvement, offer a useful analogue. Recent studies [Truax & Carkhuff, 1967] have shown that the negative effects of psychotherapy must also be taken into account. Conversely, for institutionalization, measurement must be made for that portion of the population who might show improvement.)

MEASUREMENT OF ENVIRONMENTAL CHARACTERISTICS

The positive findings reported from studies which have measured environments in terms of conceptual frameworks rather than institutional type (e.g., the relationship demonstrated between environmental change and psychological effects on institutionalized aged) suggest that studies of this order be encouraged. Current knowledge for describing institutional environments is poorly developed and techniques of assessment are almost non-existent. Further development in this area is required to delineate the specifics of the institutional structure that induce noxious effects.

Further, more attention must be given to adequate sampling of institutions catering to the aged. The majority of the studies reported in this review (aside from the mental hospitals) represent institutions of recognized quality; thus, the negative effects of institutionalization may be underestimated because of biased sampling of institutions.

STUDY RECOMMENDATIONS

This review of the literature suggest several research strategies that may yield unambiguous findings and provide the data necessary for enlightened policies.

1. Studies of personality characteristics associated with adaptation-maladaptation to institutional life suggest that further work in this area can be rewarding. If it is assumed that the majority of the aged who enter institutions have no viable alternative and that the possibility for structural change within institutions is limited, the most powerful investigative

(as well as practical) arrangement is to match individuals to particular institutional environments. (Such a step clearly must await the development of data on the psychological effects of different environments.) Current evidence suggests great individual variation in the capacity to adapt and perhaps to improve in institutional settings; it also appears that a significant proportion of the aged are clearly mismatched with respect to institutional settings and suffer serious malfunctioning and sometime death.

2. The findings from studies investigation institutionalization in terms of environmental change are also encouraging. Theory and empirical data are needed to illuminate the relations between environmental disruptions and other types of psychological losses among the aged. Specific and detailed information about the disruptiveness of environmental change could lead to ameliorative procedures to lessen the discontinuities in environment and thus the negative effects of institutionalization. Although there are anecdotal descriptions of programs preparing aged individuals for institutionalization, the lack of empirical studies comparable to studies of childhood hospitalization (Prough et al., 1963; Vaughan, 1957) is striking. The methods developed in childhood hospitalization studies considerably ameliorated the deleterious aspects of hospitalization in children; it is likely that similar results would obtain for the aged.

3. Comparative analysis of institutions offers the greatest likelihood of determining the particular institutional characteristics affecting the psychological state of the aged who enter institutions. The lack of an appreciable contribution from the current studies results from methodological difficulties that are resolvable. Longitudinal (or follow-up) studies which assessed populations prior to entering a selected cross-section of institutions would allow more precise determination of the amount and kind of influences produced by institutionalization. Some situations lend themselves more readily than others to such an approach; for example, some institutions have lists of individuals awaiting admission, which permits studying waiting-list samples. Where institutions have no waiting lists, it is feasible to identify subpopulations who tend to congregate in specific institutions (for example, in VA domiciliaries). Such a method could partially cope with the problem of economically locating institution-bound individuals prior to the actual time of institutionalization. Comparative analysis must be based on an articulated framework for viewing institutional environments and must use a similar set of measures to study institutional effects on psychological well-being. Although complex, such a research program is feasible and would provide perhaps the single most fruitful approach for providing definite information about the effects of institutional living in general and the specifics of institutional environments.

SOME THEORETICAL CONSIDERATIONS

The relative lack of communication among investigators concerned with institutionalization among children, among mentally ill, and among aged hampers the development of conceptual and technical advances. Available studies allow no firm conclusions about whether there are important differences in the effects of institutionalization on children, mentally ill persons, and aged. Comparative studies, although technically complex, might elucidate effects peculiar to aged, if any.

The psychology of aging is not adequately reflected in most of the institutional literature on the aged. Are there unique characteristics of the aged that should be considered in determining the appropriate institutional setting for such a population? The tenuous conceptual bridges between social structure and individual behavior limits understanding of behavioral effects of institutionalization on aged persons. For example, are the aged more or less reactive to environmental stimuli than younger people, or are there particular characteristics of the environment to which they are highly responsive and others to which they are less responsive? What are the expected and the acceptable environmental conditions and how do they affect the behavior of the aged as distinct from other age groups? Some information concerning the social relationships of aged persons has already been used (e.g., age-homogeneous, age-hetrogeneous) with success in studying the effects of institutionalization; utilization of the knowledge now available on the sociological and psychological aspects of aging would appreciably increase the effectiveness of such studies.

A recent review of the literature (Vernon et.al., 1965) on the effects of institutions on children vividly demonstrates the parallelism. Frequent references in studies are made to regressive behavior, lowered level of social functioning, depression. Not only are some of the psychological effects parallel to the aged, but the factors seen as causing such effects (a new and strange environment, issues of separation and sensory-motor deprivation and restriction) are similar. The problems of research are also parallel — the separation of effects of institutionalization from effects of illness, issues of particular personality characteristics associated with high risk, the effects of structural organization in institutions to ameliorate institutional effects, and the usefulness of preparation prior to institutionalization.

References

Ainsworth, M. D. *Deprivation of maternal care:* New York: Schocken Books, 1966.

Aldrich, C. K., & Mendkoff, E. Relocation of the aged and disabled: A mortality study. *Journal of the American Geriatrics Society*, 1963, **II**, 185-194.

Ames, L. B, Learned, J., Metraux, R., & Walker, R. *Rorschach responses in old age.* New York: Hoeber Harper, 1954.

Bennett, R., Nahemow, L., & Zubin, J. The effects on residents of homes for the aged on social adjustment USPHS Grant No. 0029, mimeographed progress report, 1964.

Birren, J. E. (Ed.)*Handbook of aging and the individual.* Chicago: University of Chicago Press, 1959.

Blenkner, M. Environmental change and the aging individual. *Gerontologist*, 1967, **7**, No. 2, Pt. I, 101-105.

Bortner, R. W. Test differences attributable to age selection, processes, and institutional effects. *Journal of Gerontology*, 1962, **17**, 58-60.

Camargo, O., & Preston, G. H. What happens to patients who are hospitalized for the first time when over sixty-five? *American Journal of Psychiatry*, 1945, **102**, 168-173.

Carp, F. M. The impact of environment on old people. *Gerontologist*, 1967, **7**, No. 2, Pt. I, 105-108.

Chalfen, L. Leisure-time adjustment of the aged: II. Activities and interests and some factors influencing choice. *Journal of Genetic Psychology, 1956*, **88**, 261-276.

Coe, R. M. Institutionalization and self-conception. Unpublished PhD dissertation, Washington University, St. Louis, 1962.

Davidson, H. H., & Kroglov, L. Personality characteristics of the institutionalized aged. *Journal of Consulting Psychology*, 1952, **16**, 5-12.

Dobson, W. R., & Patterson, T. W. A behavioral evaluation of geriatric patients living in nursing homes as compared to a hospitalization group. *Gerontologist*, 1961, **I**, 135-139.

Donahue, W. Impact of living arrangements on ego development in the elderly. In *Pattern of living and housing of middle aged and older people.* PHS No. 1496, 1965.

Dorken, H., Jr. Personality factors associated with paraplegia and prolonged hospitalization: A clinical note. *Canadian Journal of Psychology*, 1951, **5**, 134-137.

Eicker, W. F. Age-related differences in behavioral rigidity, level of aspiration, and adjustment in a veterans administration domiciliary population. Unpublished PhD dissertation, University of California, Los Angeles, 1959.

Epstein, L. J., & Simon, A. Alternatives to state hospitalization for geriatric mentally ill. Langley Porter Neuropsychiatric Clinics, San Francisco, 1967, dittoed paper.

Fink, H. The relationship of time perspective to age, institutionalization, and activity. *Journal of Gerontology*, 1957, **12**, 414-417.

Fogel, E. J., Swepston, E. R., Zintek, S. S., Vernier, C. N., Fitzgerald J. F., Marnocha, R. S., & Weschler, C. H. Problems of aging: Conclusions derived from two years of interdisciplinary study of domiciliary members in a veterans administration center. *American Journal of Psychiatry*, 1956, **112**, 724-730.

Fox, C. The intelligence of old indigent persons residing within and without a public home for the aged. *American Journal of Psychology*, 1950, **63**, 110-112.

Friedsam, H. J. Reactions of older persons to disaster-caused losses: An hypothesis of relative deprivation. *Gerontologist*, 1961, **1**, 34-37.

Fried, M. Grieving for a lost home. In L. J. Duhl (Ed.), *The urban condition*. New York: Basic Books, 1963.

Gitlitz, I. Morbidity and mortality in old age. Parts I-VIII. *Journal of the American Geriatrics Society*, 1956, **4**, 543-559, 708-721, 805-822, 896-908, 975-997; 1957, **5**, 32-48, 299-305.

Goffman, E. Asylums: *Essays on the social situation of mental patients and other inmates*. Garden City, N.Y.: Doubleday, 1961.

Goldfarb, A. I. Prevalence of psychiatric disorders in metropolitan old age and nursing homes. *Journal of the American Geriatrics Society*, 1962, **10**, 77-84.

Goldfarb, A. I., Shahinian, S. P., Turner, H. Death rates of relocated nursing home residents. Paper presented at the 17th annual meeting of Gerontological Society, New York, Nov., 1966.

Gottesman, L. E. Two treatment programs for the hospitalized aged. University of Michigan, Division of Gerontology, 1963, mimeographed.

Greenblatt, M., York, R. H., & Brown, E. L. (in collaboration with R. W. Hyde) *From a custodial to a therapeutic patient care in mental hospital: Exploration in social treatment*. New York: Russell Sage Foundation, 1955.

Jasnau, K. F. Individualized versus mass transfer of nonpsychotic geriatric patients from mental hospitals to nursing homes, with special reference to the death rate. *Journal of the American Geriatrics Society*, 1967, **15**, 280-284.

Kahana, E. The effects of age segregation on elderly psychiatric patients. Unpublished PhD dissertation, University of Chicago, 1968.

Kay, D., Norris, V., & Post, F. Prognosis in psychiatric disorders of the elderly. *Journal of Mental Science*, 1956, **102**, 129-140.

Kleemeier, R. W. Attitudes toward special settings for the aged. Paper presented at the International Seminar on the Social and Psychological Aspects of Aging, Berkeley, Calif., Aug., 1960.

Lakin, M. Formal characteristics of human figure drawings by institutionalized aged. *Journal of Gerontology*, 1960, **15**, 76-78.

Laverty, R. Nonresident aid—community versus institutional care for older people. *Journal of Gerontology*, 1950, **5**, 370-374.

Lawton, M., & Yaffe, S. Mortality, morbidity and voluntary change of residence. Paper presented at the meeting of the American Psychological Association, Washington, Sept., 1967.

Lepkowsky, J. R. The attitudes and adjustments of institutionalized and non-institutionalized Catholic aged. Unpublished PhD dissertation, 1954. Abstracted in *Dissertation Abstracts*, 1955, **15**, 287-288.

Lieberman, M. A. The relationship of mortality rates to entering a home for the aged. *Geriatrics*, 1961, **16**, 515-519.

Lieberman, M. A., & Lakin, M. On becoming an aged institutionalized individual. In W. Donahue, C. Tibbitts, & R. Williams (Eds.), *Social and psychological processes of aging*. New York: Atherton Press, 1963.

Lieberman, M. A., Prock, V. N., & Tobin, S. S. Psychological effects of institutionalization. *Journal of Gerontology*, 1968, **23**, 343-353.

Lieberman, M. A. Adaptation and survival under stress in the aged. USPHS Grant No. HD-00364, University of Chicago, in progress.

Lieberman, M. A., Tobin, S. S., & Slover, D. Effects of relocation on long-term geriatric patients. State of Illinois, Dept. of Mental Health Project No. 17-328, University of Chicago, in progress.

Lowenthal, M. F. *Lives in distress: The paths of the elderly to the psychiatric ward*. New York: Basic Books, 1964.

Mason, E. P. Some correlates of self-judgments of the aged. *Journal of Gerontology*, 1954, **9**, 324-337.

Miller, D., & Lieberman, M. A. The relationship of affect state adaptive reactions to stress. *Journal of Gerontology*, 1965, **20**, 492-497.

Montgomery, J. E. Living arrangements and housing of the rural aged in a central Pennsylvania community. In *Patterns of living and housing of middle aged and older people*. PHS No. 1496, 1965.

Pan, J. A comparison of factors in the personal adjustment of old people in the Protestant church homes for the aged and the old people living outside of institutions. Unpublished PhD dissertation, University of Chicago, 1950.

Pollack, M., Karp, E., Kahn, R. L., & Goldfarb, A. I. Perception of self in institutional aged subjects. I. Response patterns to mirror reflection. *Journal of Gerontology*, 1962, **17**, 405-408.

Prugh, D. G., Staub, E., Sands, H. H., Kirschbaum, R. M. & Lenihan E. A. A study of the emotional reactions of children and families to hospitalization and illness. *American Journal of Orthopsychiatry* 1953, **23**, 79-106.

Roth, M. The natural history of mental disorders in old age. *Journal of Mental Science*, 1955, **101**, 281-301.

Shrut, S. D. Attitudes toward old age and death. *Mental Hygiene*, 1958, **42**, 259-266.

Shanas, E. *Family relationships of older people*. National Opinion Research Center, University of Chicago, Health Information Foundation, Series No. 20, Oct., 1961.

Stanton, A. H., & Schwartz, N. S. *The mental hospital*. New York: Basic Books, 1954.

Stotsky, B. A. A controlled study of factors in a successful adjustment of mental patients to a nursing home. *American Journal of Psychiatry*, 1967, **123**, 1243-1251.

Swenson, W. M. Attitudes toward death in an aged population. *Journal of Gerontology*, 1961, **16**, 49-52.

Tobin, S. S., & Etigson, E. C. The effects of stress on the earliest memory. *Archives of General Psychiatry*, 1968, **4**, 435-444.

Townsend, P. *The last refuge—a survey of residential institutions and homes for the aged in England and Wales*. London: Routledge & Kegan Paul, 1962.

Truax, C. B., & Carkhuff, R. *Toward effective counseling and psychotherapy*. Chicago: Aldine Press, 1967.

Tuckman, J., & Lorge I. The effect of institutionalization on attitudes toward old people. *Journal of Abnormal (& Social) Psychology*, 1952, **47**, 337-344.

Vaughan, G. F. Children in hospitals. *Lancet*, 1957, **272**, (2), 1117-1120.

Vernon, D. T. A., Foley, J. M., Sipowicz, R. R., & Schulman, J. L. *The psychological responses of children to hospitalization and illness*. Springfield, Ill, Charles C Thomas, 1965.

Webb, M. A. Longitudinal sociopsychologic study of a randomly selected group of institutionalized veterans. *Journal of the American Geriatrics Society*, 1959, **7**, 730-740.

Whittier, J. R., & Williams, D. The coincidence of constancy of mortality figures for aged psychotic patients admitted to state hospitals. *Journal of Nervous & Mental Disease*, 1956, **124**, 618-620.

Yarrow, M. R., Blank, R., Quinn, O. W., Youmans, E. G., & Stein, J. Social psychological characteristics of old age. In J. E. Birren, R. N. Butler, S. W. Greenhouse, L. Sokoloff, & M. R Yarrow (Eds.), *Human aging*. Washington: U. S. Govt. Print. Office, 1961, PHS Publ. No. 986.

9

Dying

ROBERT S. MORISON, M.D.

The contemplation of death in the 20th century can tell us a good deal about what is right what is wrong with modern medicine. At the beginning of the century death came to about 15 percent of all newborn babies in their first year and to perhaps another 15 percent before adolescence. Nowadays fewer than 2 percent die in their first year and the great majority will live to be over 70.

Most of the improvement can be explained by changes in the numbers of deaths from infectious disease, brought about in large part by a combination of better sanitation, routine immunization and specific treatment with chemotherapeutic drugs or antibiotics. Also important, although difficult to quantify, are improvements in the individual's nonspecific resistance that are attributable to improved nutrition and general hygiene.

Infectious diseases typically attack younger people. Equally typically, although not uniformly, they either cause death in a relatively short time or disappear completely, leaving the individual much as he was before. That is what makes death from infection particularly poignant. The large number of people who used to die of infection died untimely deaths; they had not lived long enough to enjoy the normal human experiences of

FROM: *Scientific American*, Vol. 229, September 1973, pp. 55-62.

love, marriage, supporting a family, painting a picture or discovering a scientific truth.

The medical profession and the individual physician clearly had every incentive to struggle endlessly against deaths of this kind. Every triumph over an untimely death was rewarded by the high probability of complete recovery and a long, happy and productive life. No wonder the profession developed an ethic that placed a preponderant emphasis on preserving life at all costs. No wonder also that it became preoccupied with the spectacular advances in science and technology that made such triumphs possible.

Nevertheless, it is still clear that we must all die sometime. As a matter of fact, the age at which the last member of a cohort, or age class, dies is now much the same as it was in biblical times. Whereas life expectancy at birth has improved by perhaps two and half times, life expectancy at 70 has changed very little. (It is now approximately 12 years.) The difference is that in earlier times relatively few people managed to reach 70, whereas under present conditions nearly two-thirds of the population reach that age. As a result most people no longer die of some quick, acute illness but of the chronic deteriorations of old age. Only very recently has the general public or even the medical profession begun to realize that the attitudes and techniques developed in the battle against untimely death may not be entirely appropriate in helping the aged patient adapt to changed physiological and psychological circumstances.

The progress of technology puts in the physician's hands a constantly increasing number of things he can do for and to his aging patients. In the jargon of modern policy, the "options" have been greatly increased and the problem of therapy has become largely a problem of choice. Modern students of decision theory point out that all methods of choice making reduce ultimately to the making of value judgments. When a pediatrician encounters an otherwise normal child with a life-threatening sore throat, the value judgment is simple and immediate. The life is obviously worth saving at all costs and the only choice to be made is what antibiotic to use. At the other end of life, however, most patients present a varied mosaic of diminished and disordered function. For a man or woman over a certain age there is no such thing as complete recovery. Treatment directed at supporting one vital system may simply bring into greater prominence a more awkward or more painful disorder. Furthermore, many of the treatment options, unlike the treatment of acute infections that may threaten premature death, are far from simple and inexpensive. Instead they are often cumbersome, painful and costly. The art, moreover, is constantly changing, so that it is hard to estimate the probable results of some of the most elaborate procedures.

For example, in managing the course of a patient with chronic cardiovascular disease the physician has available more or less conventional drugs that can strengthen and regularize the heartbeat, reduce the accumulation of excess fluid in the tissues, moderate the blood pressure and relieve the pain of reduced circulation to the heart muscle. These results can be achieved rather simply, and such treatment has for years prolonged and enhanced the quality of the life of many people over 60. Now, however, the physician must also weigh the probable results of operations to install new heart valves, replace arteries or substitute pacemakers, all at a substantial risk to the patient's life and with the certainty of considerable pain and disability. At the end of this line is the transplantation of an entire heart, with so many risks and costs that its benefits currently tempt even the most courageous only rarely.

If the disease process leaves the heart relatively untouched and concentrates on the central nervous system, other possibilities assert themselves. Medical technology can now substitute for all the life-supporting functions of the nervous system. Tubes into either the gastrointestinal tract or a vein take the place of eating, a similar tube into the bladder takes the place of normal elimination and an artificial respirator takes the place of breathing. Various electronic devices can even keep the heart beating for weeks or months beyond its appointed time.

Thus it has come about that most therapeutic decisions for people above a certain age are not life-or-death decisions in any simple either-or sense. Inevitably the physician, the patient himself (if he is in a state to do so) or the patient's family must make more or less explicit judgments of the probable quality of the life that remains, as well as its probable length.

In this changed situation the severer critics of the medical profession go to considerable length to debunk the traditional mystery and wisdom of the physician as a decision maker. Among other things, they point out that there is nothing in the technological training of physicians that equips them to deal with questions of ethical, aesthetic or human value. Some even favor legislation removing life-or-death decisions entirely from the hands of the physician and giving them to an ombudsman or to a committee of moral philosophers.

Even the closest friends of medicine must admit that the profession has brought much of the current criticism on itself by failing to maintain the balance between the technological and the humane that characterized the best physicians from the days of Hippocrates to roughly those of Sir William Osler (1849–1919). In a way physicians have been seduced, if not actually betrayed, by their very competence. They can do a great deal for their patients at a purely technological level and at the same time they face nothing but uncertainties when they confront the ineluctable ills of the spirit. Is it any wonder they rejoice in the one and neglect the other?

I have approached the problem of terminal illness, or the dying patient, in this somewhat circuitous fashion in order to show that the problems surrounding the deathbed are not quite so unprecedented or so unconnected with the rest of medicine as to require the development of entirely new attitudes or perhaps even a new profession of "thanatologists." Dying is continuous with living, and the questions that are now asked with such insistence at the bedside of the dying should also be at least in the back of the mind of those who attend the living in earlier stages. The physician must consider the quality of the life he is struggling to preserve and the probable effects of his therapy on this quality, whatever the age of the patient. He should also know how to help a patient of any age to accept circumstances that cannot be changed. The so-called terminally ill patient simply represents the limiting case. In this instance the value questions have become paramount.

For reasons that are not all easy to identify the past few years have seen an astonishing increase in public attention to death and dying. A recent bibliography listing the titles of both books and papers in scholarly journals on the subject is several pages long. It is a rare daily newspaper or popular periodical that has not published one such article or several. Approaches to the topic may be roughly separated into two classes: those that deal with making the patient's last days as physically and psychologically comfortable as possible and those that discuss the propriety of allowing or helping the patient to die at an appropriate time. Let us turn first to the care of the terminally ill.

Students of the process of dying have long emphasized the loneliness of the dying person. Not only is he destined to go where no one wants to follow but also the people around him prefer to pretend that the journey is really not going to take place. The practice of placing familiar articles and even animals, servants and wives in the tomb or on the funeral pyre of the departed is testimony to man's desire to assuage the loneliness beyond. In "The Death of Ivan Ilych" Leo Tolstoy has given the classic description of the conspiracy of denial that so often surrounds the dying. The situation has certainly been made worse by the technological changes since Tolstoy's day. Then, at least, most people died at home, many of them surrounded by family and friends. Even if these attendants were primarily concerned with what would happen to themselves, as were those awaiting the death of the old Count Bezhukoi that Tolstoy also portrayed, they not only kept the patient from being physically alone but also made him quite conscious of being the center of attention.

Nowadays only a minority of people die at home, and the number is decreasing. Precise figures are hard to obtain, but the scattered studies that have been made agree that about half of all deaths occur in large general hospitals and a smaller but increasing number in nursing homes. Probably fewer than a third die at home, at work or in public places.

The past few years have seen a growing awareness that the big general hospital is not a very good place to die. Even though such hospitals have large staffs, most of these professionals are preoccupied with administrative matters and with the increasingly complicated technical aspects of keeping people alive. Surrounded by these busybodies, the dying patient is more often than not psychologically isolated. Recognizing that such an atmosphere is bad both for patients and for youngster physicians in training, a few inspired physicians have developed special programs to instruct members of the hospital staff in the needs of the dying patient. Such efforts have been received with enthusiasm by the still quite limited numbers of physicians and students who have been exposed to them.

The usefulness of training hospital staff members to deal with the dying patient is a concept that is now spreading throughout the country. There is substantial hope that the next generation of physicians, nurses and administrators will be much more understanding and helpful in meeting the special needs of the dying than their predecessors were. One of the leaders in this movement is an Illinois psychiatrist, Elisabeth K. Ross. In an effort to inject something approaching methodological rigor into her understanding and teaching of the needs of the dying, she has distinguished five stages exhibited by dying patients: denial, anger, bargaining (usually with God), depression and acceptance. This effort toward intellectualization of the problem is admirable; at the same time it is probably true that what has been most influential in alleviating the loneliness of the dying is the warmth of Dr. Ross's sympathy and the intensity of her dedication to the effort.

A high proportion of the patients in nursing homes are destined to die there or to be removed only at the very last minute for intensive hospital care, yet few of these institutions appear to have given much thought to the special problems of the dying. The most striking exceptions are provided by what in England are called "hospices." The best-known of them is St. Christopher's, outside London. It was started by a physician who was also trained as a nurse. She appears to have combined the best of both professions in developing arrangements for taking care of seriously ill patients and providing a warm and understanding atmosphere for them. Because many of the patients at St. Christopher's suffer from malignant disease, special emphasis is put on the alleviation of pain. It has been found that success depends not only on providing the right drugs at the right time but also on developing an attitude of understanding, confidence and hope. Psychological support involves, among other things, deinstitutionalizing the atmosphere by encouraging members of the family, including children and grandchildren, both to "visit the patient" in a formal sense and to carry on such activities as may be usual for their age, so that the patient feels surrounded by ongoing normal life. Everyone who has observed the program or has been privileged to participate in it speaks appreciatively and even enthusiastically about its achievements.

Hospices also serve as centers for an active home-care program that is demonstrating the practicality of tending to many dying patients in the home, provided that the physical arrangements are satisfactory and that specialized help from outside is available for a few hours a day. Unfortunately most insurance plans, including the otherwise enlightened National Health Service in Britain, have tended to emphasize hospital care to the detriment of adequate support for proper care in the home.

Recent studies of home care for seriously ill patients suggest that in many cases it can be not only more satisfactory emotionally than hospital care but also considerably less costly. Much more information is needed before administrators of health plans can determine precisely how many and what kinds of personnel should be available for how long to deal with various kinds of home situation. Similarly, a few preliminary surveys of the technological ways of adapting the American home for the care of the chronically ill have been made. Here again there is enough information to suggest the importance of funds for special types of beds and wheelchairs, the installation of plumbing within easy range of the sickbed and so on. The data, however, are not yet precise enough to allow adequate planning or the calculation of insurance premiums adequate to cover such services.

In spite of the potential emotional and economic benefits of home care one cannot overlook the fact that many social and technological changes have made illness and death at home very different from what they were in the days of Ivan Ilych and Count Bezhukoi. It is not appropriate here to try to cast up an account of the costs and benefits of such factors as rising social and geographic mobility and the transition from the extended family to the nuclear family. When these costs are counted, however, it may be well to include mention of the increasing difficulty in finding a good place to grow old and die.

Let us next examine the question of when it becomes appropriate to die. No matter how considerate the physician, how supportive the institutional atmosphere, how affectionately concerned the family and friends or how well-adjusted the patient himself, there comes a time when all those involved must ask themselves just how much sense it makes to continue vigorously trying to postpone the inevitable. Regrettably the literature addressed to the topics of death and dying often seems preoccupied more with dissecting the various ethical and legal niceties surrounding the moment and manner of death than with what one can do to make the last few months or years of life as rewarding as possible. No doubt this preoccupation is prompted by an apparent conflict between ancient taboos on the one hand and certain obvious commonsense considerations on the other.

Now, virtually no one who has thought about the matter at all, from John Doe to the Pope, feels that any absolute moral or legal obligation requires one to do everything one knows how to do in order to preserve the life of a severely deteriorated patient beyond hope of recovery. Indeed, in actual practice it now seems probable that only a small minority of patients have everything possible done for them right up to the moment of death. The difficulties, then, are not with the general principle but with how to arrange the details. First and foremost in presenting themselves are the theoretical and even metaphysical problems involved in the ways that men of goodwill attempt to justify actions that appear to violate the taboo against killing. Second, there are practical questions to be answered. How can the individual make sure that his wishes are carried out? Who is to make the decision if the patient is no longer competent to do so? What are the physician's responsibilities? What, for that matter, are his possible liabilities? How far should society go in attempting to protect the rights and regulate the behavior of the various parties?

No more than an outline of the theoretical problems can be presented here. Current discussion centers principally on three issues. First is the definition of death. Next is the difference, if any, between negative and positive euthanasia and last is the definition of "extraordinary means."

The possibility of redefining death came into prominence a few years ago when a group of Boston physicians grew concerned about precisely when it was appropriate to remove a prospective donor's organs for transplantation. It rapidly became clear that "defining" death, for whatever purpose, is a complicated philosophical matter that admits of no easy resolution. What the members of the Boston group actually did was to devise an operational redefinition of the criteria to be applied in declaring that a person has died. The major difficulty they faced arose from the purely technical fact that it is now possible to maintain the function of the heart and the lungs by artificial means. The failure of these two vital functions can therefore no longer be regarded in all cases as the paramount criteria for pronouncing death, as was once set forth in all conventional medical-legal texts.

The Boston group instead recommended the use of a set of signs testifying to an essentially complete failure of a third set of functions: those of the nervous system. This proposal has been received with approval by a large number of physicians, theologians and lawyers, and has now been included in the law of several states. The criteria as they stand are extremely rigid and involve the death of essentially all levels of the nervous system. They thus seem entirely adequate both to protect the patient against premature assaults in order to retrieve viable organs and at the same time to guard him against unduly zealous attempts to maintain elementary vital signs in the name of therapy.

There is another class of patients, however, in whom elementary vital signs have not failed, although the higher brain functions—thinking, communicating with others and even consciousness itself—have departed. Such a patient constitutes a most distressing problem to families and physicians, and it has been suggested that a further revision of the criteria for a pronouncement of death might be used to justify the termination of active treatment in such cases. The idea is that what is really human and important about the individual resides in the upper levels of the nervous system, and that these attributes indeed die with the death of the forebrain.

The presumed merit of such a revision grows out of the way it avoids the basic ethical problem; obviously it makes no sense to go on treating what can rationally be defined as a corpse. The weight of opinion, however, seems to be against dealing with the question of cerebral incapacity in this oblique way. From several standpoints it seems preferable to face up to the fact that under these circumstances a patient may still be living in some sense, but that the obligation to treat the living is neither absolute nor inexorable.

No less a moral authority than the Pope appears to have lent his weight to this view and even to have spoken for most Christians when he announced a few years ago that the physician is not required to use "extraordinary means" to maintain the spark of life in a deteriorated patient with no evident possibility of recovery. Nevertheless, serious ambiguities still remain. At first the Vatican's phraseology appears to have been designed to allow the withdrawal of "heroic" and relatively novel procedures such as defibrillation, cardiac massage and artificial respiration. More subtle analysts point out that there is no absolute scale of extraordinariness, and that what is or is not extraordinary can only be judged in relation to the condition of a given individual. Hence there is nothing extraordinary about using all possible means to keep alive a young mother who has suffered multiple fractures, severe hemorrhages and temporary unconsciousness. Conversely, the term extraordinary may well be applied to relatively routine procedures such as intravenous feeding if the patient is elderly, has deteriorated and has little hope of improvement. Thus the most active proponents of the doctrine of extraordinary means clearly interpret "extraordinary" to mean "inappropriate in the circumstances." Although many people who hold this position would disagree, it is not easy for an outsider to distinguish their interpretation from advocacy of what is sometimes called "negative euthanasia."

Negative euthanasia refers to withdrawal of treatment from a patient who as a result is likely to die somewhat earlier than he otherwise would. Many thoughtful and sensitive people who favor the principle dislike the term because it suggests that treatment is being withdrawn with an actual, if unspoken, intent to shorten the patient's life. These critics, who place a high value on the taboo against taking life, prefer to regard the withdrawal of active therapy as simply a matter of changing from a therapeutic regime that is inappropriate to one that is more appropriate under the circumstances. If death then supervenes, it is not regarded as the result of anything the physician has or has not done but simply as a consequence of the underlying illness. Thus the physician and those who have perhaps participated in his decision are protected from the fear that they are "playing God" or from similar feelings of guilt.

Many of those who favor negative euthanasia also recognize that appropriate care of the terminally ill may include "positive" procedures, such as giving morphine (which, among other effects, may advance the moment of death). Invoking what is known in Catholic circles as the doctrine, or law, of double effect, they regard such positive actions as permissible as long as the conscious intent is to achieve some licit purpose such as the relief of pain. This view in turn requires the drawing of an important moral distinction between "awareness of probable result" and "intent."

Other moralists, such as the blunter and more forthright proponents of what is called situational ethics, may dismiss such subtleties as irrelevant logic-chopping. In their view it is a mistake to extend the generalized taboos and abstract principles of the past to encompass the peculiarities of the 20th-century death scene. They prefer to focus attention on the scene itself and to do what seems best in terms of the probable results for all concerned. Perhaps not surprisingly, the situational ethicist, who derives much of his philosophical base from classical utilitarian, or consequential, ethics, sees relatively little difference between negative and positive euthanasia, that is, between allowing to die and causing to die.

For the sake of completeness let me inject my own opinion that although there may be only a trivial intellectual distinction between negative and positive euthanasia, it seems unwise and in any event useless at this time to enter into an elaborate defense of positive euthanasia. Although the principle has its enthusiastic advocates, their number is strictly limited. The overwhelming majority of physicians and certainly a substantial majority of laymen instinctively recoil from such active measures as prescribing a known poison or injecting a large bubble into a vein. There seems to be a point where simple human reactions supersede both legal sanction and rational analysis. As an example, very few New York physicians or nurses are anxious to exercise the right given them by the laws of the state to perform abortions as late as the 24th week of pregnancy.

Furthermore, it appears that as a practical matter negative euthanasia, or the withdrawal of all active therapy except the provision of narcotics to subdue restlessness and pain, will in any case be followed in a reasonable length of time by the coming of what Osler termed near the turn of the century the "old man's friend": a peaceful death from bronchial pneumonia. Thus, in the terminology of the law courts, we need not reach the most difficult question.

In view of the prevailing theoretical uncertainties, it is not surprising that what is done to or for the dying patient varies widely from place to place and from physician to physician. It is impossible to be precise because very few scientific observations have been made. Perhaps the most careful study is one conducted by Diana Crane of the University of Pennsylvania, who asked a large number of physicians and surgeons what they would probably do in a series of precisely outlined clinical situations. From this and more anecdotal evidence it seems clear that very few do everything possible to prolong the lives of all their patients. At the other extreme, even fewer physicians would appear to employ active measures with the avowed intent of shortening life. In between there is an enormous range of decisions: to give or not to give a transfusion, to prescribe an antibiotic or a sulfa drug, to attach or disconnect a respirator or an artificial kidney, to install a cardiac pacemaker to let the battery of one that is already installed run down. The overall impression gained both by the informed observer and by the sometimes despairing layman is that the median of all these activities lies rather far toward officiously keeping alive.

The reasons are obvious enough: the momentum of a professional tradition of preserving life at all costs, the reluctance of the physician and the layman to ignore ancient taboos or to impair the value of such positive concepts as the sanctity of life, and the ambiguities of the love-hate relationship between parents and children or husbands and wives. Finally, there is the continuing uncertainty about the legal position of a physician who might be charged with hastening the death of a patient by acts of either omission or commission.

Up to now, at least, the legal deterrent appears to have been something of a chimera. A conscientious search of the available literature in English has uncovered not one criminal action charging that a physician omitted treatment with the intent to shorten life. Indeed, there are surprisingly few actions that charge positive euthanasia. Even in the few actions that have been lodged, juries have shown a reluctance to convict when there is evidence that the action was undertaken in good faith to put the patient on the far side of suffering.

Approaching the problem from a somewhat different angle, although the definitive examples are few, there appears to be general agreement that the adult patient in full possession of his senses has every right to refuse treatment. It is somewhat less certain that such refusal is binding after a patient loses legal competence. Even less clear is the status of the expressed wish of a potential patient with respect to what he would want done in certain hypothetical future circumstances. Efforts to clarify the status of such communications, sometimes called "living wills," with physicians and relatives are being actively pursued.

Important though it may be to establish the rights and privileges of those foresighted enough to want to participate in the design of their own death, it must be admitted that such individuals now constitute only a trivial part of the population. The great majority prefer not to think about their own death in any way. Indeed, most people do not even leave a will directing what to do with their material possessions.

What, then, can be done for that large number of people likely to slip into an unanticipated position of indignity on a deathbed surrounded by busybodies with tubes and needles in their hands, ready to substitute a chemical or mechanical device for every item in the human inventory except those that make human life significant? In such instances, under ideal, or perhaps I should say idyllic, circumstances the attending physician would have known the patient and his family for a long time. Further, he would have sensed their conscious and unconscious wishes and needs, and drawing on his accumulated skills and wisdom, he would conduct the last illness so as to maximize the welfare of all concerned. Unfortunately under modern conditions few families have a regular physician of any kind and even fewer physicians possess the hypothetical virtues I have outlined.

However that may be, at least three approaches to the problem are being actively pursued at present. Foremost among them is the active discussion I have referred to. Not only the professional journals but also the monthly, weekly and daily press are publishing numerous articles on death and dying. Radio and television programs have followed suit, and it must be a rare church discussion group that has not held at least one meeting devoted to death with dignity. At the very least such discussion must remove some of the reluctance to speak of death or even think about it. At best it must improve the possibility of communication and understanding between the patient and the physician. The resulting change in the climate of opinion cannot fail to make it easier to discard outmoded taboos in favor of the common sense of contemporary men.

Second, and equally important, are the formal and informal efforts to improve the education of physicians by redressing the imbalance between technical skill and human wisdom that has grown up during the present century. In addition to the kind of clinical concern for the dying exemplified by Dr. Ross, many medical schools are converting their courses in medical ethics from a guild-oriented preoccupation with fee splitting and other offenses against the in-group to a genuine concern for ethical values in the treatment of patients.

Third, there are the more formal attempts to clarify rights, responsibilities and roles by means of legislation. Part of this effort is directed at establishing the obligation of a physician to follow the expressed wishes of his patient or, at the very least, at protecting the physician from liability if he does so. Other legislative proposals stem from a more or less explicit conviction that death is too important a matter to be left to physicians. Difficulty is often encountered, however, in finding a satisfactory alternative, and there is now much discussion of the relative merits of assigning ultimate authority to the next-of-kin, to an ombudsman or to a committee of social scientists, philosophers and theologians.

It is too early to predict how such suggestions will turn out, but there are some reasons for feeling that it may be well to go slow in formalizing what is bound to be a difficult situation and instead to redouble efforts toward developing the capacity of medical men and laymen to deal informally with the problem. In actual practice the conduct of a drawn-out terminal illness involves a series of small decisions, based on repeated evaluations of the physical and emotional condition of the patient and the attitudes, hopes and fears of his family and friends. It is not easy to see how an outsider such as an ombudsman, much less a committee, can be very easily fitted into what is typically an unobtrusive incremental process. Concrete evidence on this point may be found with respect to the beginning of life in the attempts by opponents of contraception to inject either a sheriff or a bureaucrat, so to speak, into the bedroom. These attempts have not proved satisfactory and are more and more being denounced by the courts as invasions of privacy.

As long as progress is being made at the informal, grass-roots level, it may be just as well to refrain from drafting tidy legislative solutions to problems so profound. Whatever else may be said, it is obvious that changing attitudes toward death and dying provide an excellent paradigm of how changing technologies force on us the consideration of equally significant changes in value systems and social institutions.

CHAPTER 4

SYSTEMS

Systems, systems approach, systems analysis, systems design, and other systems-related terms and concepts are being used increasingly in management, engineering, health, social sciences, and many other disciplines.

A system is a set of interrelated and interdependent parts designed to achieve a set of goals. This definition of the term "system," although brief, has widespread and far-reaching implications. Not many entities, be they concrete or abstract, consist of less than two parts.*As such, anything that is the focus of our attention can be viewed as a system. All human activities relate to and deal with systems. There are social systems, business systems, political systems, health-care systems, long-term care systems, and so on. Within a long-term care facility, there are patient-care systems, information systems, financial systems and other related systems. A hierarchy of systems can thus be created,

---

*Obviously not all entities have delineated, specified, desire goals. Nor are all entities capable of achieving their goals — because of internal conflicts and external disturbances. Accordingly, in real life, both systems and non-systems coexist simultaneously.

depending upon the nature, scope, and purpose of the systems study.

The major function of any health-care system is to achieve an optimal level of health for a defined population through the delivery of comprehensive health programs. It is clear that long-term care is a necessary component of comprehensive health care, although it has frequently been ignored in planning for comprehensive care systems. Long-term care can be, and must be, viewed as a subsystem of the overall health system. Only in this manner can rational health planning be undertaken at different levels in society and among different types of health-care organizations.

Management is the primary force that coordinates the activities of the subsystems of an organization and relates them to the environment.* In the health services, as in any field of human endeavor, the effectiveness with which individuals work together toward the achievement of goals and objectives in their man-made social systems, called organizations, is principally a function of the level of managerial competence. Managers must be prepared to understand the forces at work in organizational situations and to exercise control over them where it is appropriate.

Recognition of the requisite for upgrading the efficiency and effectiveness of management performance in all health organizations, including long-term care facilities, is partly a reflection of the complexities and accelerating rate of change inherent in modern society. It is also to a large extent a function of the realization that availability and accessibility of resources are necessary, but not sufficient, conditions for the improved organization and delivery of health care and that applications of the systems concept to the health field should be stimulated. The report of the *National Advisory Commission on Health Manpower* indicated that the crisis in health care was not simply a crisis of numbers. They state that, "It is true that substantially increased numbers of health manpower will be needed over time. But if additional personnel are employed in the present manner and within the present patterns and 'Systems' of care, they will not avert, or even perhaps alleviate, the crisis. *Unless we improve the*

---

*Johnson, R.A., Kast, F.E., and Rosenzweig, J.E., The Theory and Management of Systems, New York: Mc-Graw-Hill Book Company, 1967, p. 14.

system through which health care is provided, care will continue to become less satisfactory, even though there are massive increases in cost and numbers of health personnel."* Improvement of the total health system in a general sense is a direct function of the extent to which the management of the system can be enhanced.

The role of systems theory for the manager is to enable him to reach better levels of understanding of complex organizations. Unfortunately, organizational systems are difficult to define because they are not measurable physical entities. Organizations are ubiquitous phenomena in which we spend a considerable proportion of our lives in one capacity or another. They provide for the needs of the individual in many areas, and long-term care is no exception. Furthermore, organizations engaged in the delivery of health care are highly complex, dynamic systems that undergo a continuous interaction with a wide array of political, economic, social, and technological forces.

The term "systems" is one that is frequently misunderstood and misused. BUCKLEY (Selection 10) points out that the term is one of the most common in our vocabulary. It is also ambiguous and this often leads to abuses of systems concepts which, in turn, hinders efforts to design, operate, and evaluate systems. The author distinguishes between two broad uses of the word "systems" as it is used in "general systems theory" and "operating systems theory." *General systems theory* is an approach to the observation and solution of problems which considers each alternative solution as a cost-benefit relationship. Each solution therefore has a cost as well as a benefit. The more realistic method then is to seek an option which has the lowest relative cost and the highest benefit. While the emphasis in general systems theory is on the *framework of the problem,* in *operating systems theory* the emphasis is on the *medium* of problem-solving (e.g., accounting). Buckley underscores the necessity for understanding the import of three related terms — "system," "goal," and "process." Together these merge into a cohesive theoretic structure called GPS (Goal, Process, Systems). Three forms of the GPS complex are

---

Report of the National Advisory Commission on Health Manpower, Vol. 1, Washington, D.C.: U.S. Government Printing Ofice, November 1967, p. 2.

described. The author discusses the properties of goals, processes, and systems. He concludes the article with a recognition and examination of the reality that the ultimate objective in management is to reach goals in the most efficient manner. This is possible only in the context of systems and process data, but unfortunately the latter have been meager in relation to the former. This is equally true in the long-term care institution.

DOLGOFF (Selection 11) deals with a much neglected but vital aspect of health and long-term care management: namely, the administration of mental health facilites. The approach that is assumed in this analysis is largely behavioral, and the author attempts to integrate concepts derived from industrial settings with mental health administration. Dolgoff notes the importance of organizational, personality, and interpersonal factors in socio-technical systems and provides an analysis of those separate subsystems in a psychiatric hospital. He illustrates the ramifications of several types of organizational conflict through an excerpt from an administrative report. The common consequences of role conflict, tension, and anxiety that result in cognitive, emotional, and physiological responses that vary in intensity and duration are recognized. Administrators and professionals often hold differing views of what work will be undertaken, how it will be accomplished, when, and, by whom. In the long-term care institution, organizational conflict can be reduced through an understanding of the complexity and diversity of goals, norms, values, incentives, and power strategies.

BROWN (Selection 12) presents the main components of general systems theory. The term "system" is defined and some basic concepts and characteristics of systems are presented. Three basic system characteristics relevant to organizations are *flows, structure,* and *procedures.* A distinction is made between a *closed* and an *open* system. Organizations can best be understood if they are viewed and managed as open systems that affect, and are affected by their environment. Long-term care institutions are open systems to the extent that they draw energy from the outside, store resources for possible future crises, and maintain a dynamic balance. The article concludes by listing a set of limitations and criticisms of the systems approach to organizational and managerial problems.

GROSS (Selection 13) emphasizes the need for the *systems approach* in planning and developing organization objectives. The organization is *not* a single-purpose entity. The performance and structure of any organization have multiple dimensions which must be integrated and reconciled by developing a "general-system model" of an organization. Gross describes such a model by enumerating seven activities that describe the dimensions of performance and seven organizational components that define structure.

10

Goal-Process-System
Interaction in Management

JOHN W. BUCKLEY

Most of us were introduced to this word "systems" at an early age. We learned of school systems, the solar system, and other elementary systems, and this vocabulary grew as our education progressed. We learned of physiological, transportation, political, and planning and control systems, and the systems approach. Clearly, the term is one of the most ubiquitous in our vocabulary.

Unfortunately, the meaning of "systems" is also shrouded in ambiguity. Ask for a succinct definition of the word, and you will be surprised at the vagueness of the answers. Those with more exposure to systems theory couch their ambiguity in such expressions as "interconnected networks of interrelated entities," leaving themselves and their listeners with uneasiness as to the meaning of the word.

This ambiguity leads to abuse of systems concepts and hinders our efforts to design, operate, and evaluate systems. But the notion of a system is so basic and so potentially useful that we should try to clarify it.

TWO GENERAL USES

We can distinguish at once between two broad uses of the word as it is used in general systems theory and in operating systems theory.

FROM: *Business Horizons*, December 1971, pp. 81-92.

General systems theory refers to a way or approach by which to observe and solve problems. Because of its emphasis on the way problems are tackled, it is often referred to as the systems aproach, or, more viscerally, as "organized common sense." The systems approach insists on the broadest possible understanding of a problem, involves exploring all feasible alternatives, and selects the best solution through rational means.

To illustrate the systems approach, consider the problem of meeting the demand for more electricity. A search for feasible alternatives begins. Long-range solutions provide more flexibility in that they allow us to consider alternatives which may not be feasible at present. If the need is immediate, our search is bounded by the existing state of technology.

There are basically three means for generating electricity at present: hydroelectric power, the use of hydrocarbons such as coal or oil, and nuclear power. Feasibility involves technological, economic, and social considerations. There are pros and cons to each alternative. While hydroelectric power plants produce "clean" electricity at relatively low cost, there are not enough suitable sites for dams, and the distances to major user areas are too great. A new social cost has been added recently in the destruction of scenic river beds. Conventional power plants using coal or oil produce smog and other contaminants, and are inefficient in converting hydrocarbons into electric power. Nuclear plants are more efficient, but the problem of thermal pollution and the fear of accidents weigh heavily on the negative scale.

In the language of general systems theory, every alternative is a cost-benefit relationship. Thus, it is not practical to think of zero-cost solutions, but rather to seek the option which has the lowest relative cost and highest benefit. (This may involve a combination of alternatives.) In our example, a decision not to pollute the air may necessitate a decision to pollute the water. A final decision of this type is often made in the social arena.

Suppose that perfect data are available that lead us to favor nuclear plants for technoeconomic reasons. While our problem may appear to be solved in quantitative terms, the systems approach requires that we go further, for even good theoretic solutions may fail for want of public acceptance.

The systems approach requires us to consult public opinion. If it is favorable, implementation can proceed, but if it is opposed, it is necessary either to change public opinion or to choose a less optimal strategy.

In those instances where the best solution involves a technology which has no operating history, the systems approach calls for testing under real-world conditions. These simulations provide decision makers with real instead of theoretical data and reduce the risks of choosing and implementing faulty solutions.

To summarize, some fundamentals of general systems theory are as follows: (1) it proposes a structured approach to problem solving; (2) its methodology is explicit, which means that there are guidelines to problem solving; (3) the boundaries of a problem are identified; (4) all feasible solutions are measured in terms of cost-benefit; and (5) the best solution in the light of technical, economic, and social considerations is adopted.

Operating systems theory involves a second broad use of the term systems. Here the meaning is different from the meaning of the term when used in general systems theory, where systems is synonymous with a particular problem-solving framework. When we speak of a transportation, an accounting, or a weapons delivery system, we do not think of a methodology or approach, but of a functioning medium through which actions are undertaken.

We can achieve a better understanding of systems in the operational sense by placing it in a context with two other concepts with which it is closely related. These related terms are "goal" and "process"; with "system," they form a cohesive theoretic structure which we will call a GPS Complex.

A goal is an objective, a desired attainment. It answers the question "why" and explains the reason for an action. A process is a set of prescribed activities or strategies by which we attain goals. It answers the question "what is happening" and defines the essence of an activity. A system is the network of resources needed to perform the activity. It answers the question "how" and describes the mechanics that allow processes to occur.

The logic of the GPS Complex can be illustrated by an example from physiology, where the goal (satisfaction of the hunger need) is achieved by the process (eating) through a system (a network of resource elements which enable us to eat, such as food, utensils, heat and cold, and so on). We observe that goals cannot be reached without processes, and that processes cannot take place without systems.[1]

Another observation is appropriate at this point. Our options increase as we move downward through the GPS Complex. Having asserted a goal, we have no option but to fulfill it, to abandon it, or to modify it in favor of a new goal. However, given a goal, a limited choice exists as to processes. In our example, the hunger need could be "satisfied" in a limited number of ways. An alternative to eating would be surgery to remove the hunger-

---

[1] Robert Anthony, *Planning and Control Systems: a Framework for Analysis* (Cambridge: Harvard University Press, 1965), p. 5, distinguishes between processes and systems in these words: "In brief, a system facilitates a process; it is the means by which processes occur. The distinction is similar to that between anatomy and physiology. Anatomy deals with structure—what it is; whereas physiology deals with process—how it functions. The digestive system facilitates the process of digestion."

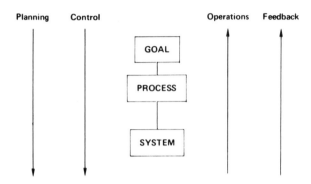

FIGURE 1. Management Flows Through the GPS Complex

inducing impulses, or a process by which mental control is exercised over the physical urge. Moving to the systems level, however, we find that alternatives are numerous, as illustrated by the many possible resource combinations for satisfying hunger.

The GPS Complex has other implications for management planning and control as shown in Figure 1. Effective planning is possible only as we move from known goals to the definition of processes and the design of systems. Hence the flow is downward through the GPS Complex. Similarly, controls flow from goals; their purpose is to assure that activities conform to plans.

Operations, on the other hand, begin at the systems level, generating an activity flow that culminates in results (achieved goals). Feedback also originates at the systems level in the form of reports on the level of activity, on exceptions, on the functioning of controls, and the interpretation of events.

GPS STRUCTURES

The GPS Complex assumes many different forms. These can be grouped under the three basic types shown in Figure 2.

Type A Structure

In Type A, each element is related exclusively to the other elements. For example, to meet the goal of telling time, we have the time-keeping process, and the system element is a watch. Unless the watch also serves

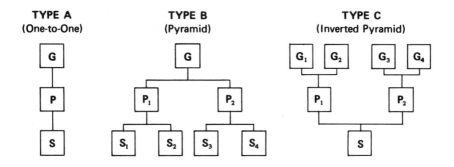

FIGURE 2. Three Basic Types of GPS Complex

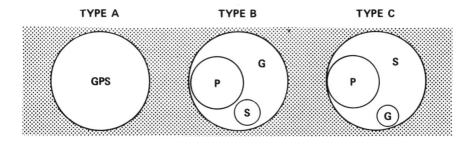

FIGURE 3. GPS Elements in Three Basic Structures

some other objective, such as decoration, its sole function is to enable us to tell time through the process of timekeeping. In the language of set theory, the elements G, P, and S occupy contiguous areas in the Type A structure (Figure 3).

Compared with Types B and C, Type A is relatively easy to design and operate. Cost-benefit analysis is aided in that there are no shared systems costs or process benefits.

Type B Structure

In Type B the whole focus of the structure is on a single important (and usually complex) goal, for example, the task of getting man to the moon and back. A goal like this requires several processes and many systems. Each process and system is a necessary but not a sufficient factor in reaching the goal. Processes must be combined with other processes, and systems with other systems in order to reach the objective; hence, we have an interdependency between processes and between systems. In terms of set theory, Type B structure consists of a hierarchy of importance in the order G, P, and S, as shown in Figure 3.

The pyramid is characterized by its sensitivity. As in the marble games we play, removal of one supporting element leads to the collapse of the whole structure. Also, it is difficult to add new elements after the initial design without destroying it's symmetry. Major modifications call for redesign of the structure as a whole. Managing a pyramid requires a holistic approach; each part must be viewed in terms of its impact on the whole. Because of the sensitive interdependencies between the elements, network techniques such as PERT are useful management tools.

The singular advantage of the pyramid is that all energy is directed toward one goal. This has both behavioral and economic implications. The behavioral implication is that employees in a pyramid have a discernible goal (motivator) and can measure their contribution towards its attainment. From an economic viewpoint, it is relatively easy to calculate the final cost of achieving a goal because there are no shared costs at the goal level.

The pyramid is typical of most projects and is also found in new organizations, which often begin with a single major purpose but transform progressivley into the inverted pyramid form. This transformation gives rise to behavioral and economic problems which we will discuss.

Type C Structure

Because many of our major organizations are of the inverted pyramid form, we need to study and understand them if we are to prevent the organizational senility that now appears inevitable. This structure is one large system with many goals and fewer processes. It is typical of large organizations, particularly of government, where multiple goals are financed through one large revenue collection system (IRS).

In the Type C structure, a goal is a necessary but not a sufficient reason for having the underlying process, and, similarly, a process is a necessary but not a sufficient reason for the existence of the system. In other words, a system serves a number of processes, and a process serves a number of goals. A set theory view of the "inverted pyramid" would show S as occupying the area of most importance, ranging from P to G, as shown in Figure 3.

The inverted pyramid is characterized by its insensitivity and impersonality. If we remove a goal, we cannot remove the underlying elements because they serve other goals as well. Removing goals creates redundance (unused capacity) with its attendant economic costs. On the other hand, if we keep adding goals we increasingly strain (overload) the underlying processes and systems. Because there is no direct linkage between goals and the supporting elements, there is a tendency to think in terms of goals without concern for their impact on the process-system elements.

We referred earlier to the economic and behavioral problems that are inherent in the inverted pyramid. The economic problem is posed by the difficulty of tracing costs. Since process and system costs are shared among many goals, it is difficult to know the cost of reaching a particular goal. At best, we have to rely on fairly arbitrary devices for allocating costs.

The behavioral problem arises from the intrinsic impersonality of the inverted pyramid. Employees, who form part of the systems network, have difficulty in relating to multiple goals, some of which are in conflict with each other. Therefore, preservation of the system becomes a goal in its own right.

We mentioned the typical transformation of pyramids into inverted pyramids. A scenario of this metamorphosis might run as follows. A single, visible goal gives way to many goals that become more obscure and meaningless. Employees are progressively isolated from the goal orientation of the organization. Altruistic motivation gives way to self-interest, and performance becomes competitive. Self-interest progresses into fear and insecurity, and pronounced efforts are made to obtain insularity and invulnerability per the organization itself. Efforts toward change are viewed as personal threats. In lieu of extraorganization (social) goals, the major goal becomes one of sustaining the system and making it impervious to attack. Lacking social motivation, the organization progressively fails.

Investment behavior also illustrates the transformation of a pyramid into an inverted pyramid. A new firm appeals to investors on the basis of social goals: it intends to provide goods or services that will have social (and hence economic) appeal. COMSAT is a case in point. There were many years of active trading in COMSAT stock before it launched its first satellite. In such a case, there is no history of earnings. Generally, the financial statements reveal minimal collateral in the event of failure. What then are investors buying? Simply stated, they are sharing a dream; they believe in the basic purpose of the firm.

When an organization inverts, however, investors too lack knowledge or association with its goals. The stock market now pulses on earnings and other internal data rather than on exogenous factors. Somewhere in the process of changing its GPS structure, the dream is lost.

PROPERTIES OF G, P, AND S

Goals

Goals are assertive. They are stated objectives. I can assert a goal; you can assert a goal. Some goals are more important than others because they are based in part on who makes the assertion and the willingness of others to accept his goal. Rank, the art of persuasion, access to media, and many other factors improve one's position to assert goals on behalf of others.

Goals are neutral. They are not intrinsically right or wrong. What makes some good and others bad is determined by existing social values. A good goal at one time may be a bad one at another if the value set has changed in the interval. For example, in 1960 President John F. Kennedy announced the goal of sending a "man to the moon and back within the decade." In the social climate of 1960 this was viewed by most of us as a good goal. The same objective articulated in 1971 might have far less acceptance.

This fact makes it necessary for goalsetters to tap the social mainstream constantly if they are to set forth goals which will have general acceptance. Unfortunately, this need is frustrated by the increasing insularity of higher offices.

Goals may be implicit or explicit. The confusion that results when we attempt to define the goals of government indicates that many of our large organizations function without explicit goals, by which we mean higher level or external goals as opposed to internal goals, such as improving efficiency or earnings. Yet each system is producing results (which we will call achieved goals), so that failure to articulate goals does not imply their nonexistence.

Where goals are not explicit we can deduce them by observing the system at work. This is a poor substitute for explicit goals in that the ability and resources of observers differ widely, leading to different conclusions as to the goals in question. The story of the four blind men and the elephant comes to mind. Each concluded it was a different creature because he was able to feel only a small part of the elephant's body. Making goals explicit raises the level of argument to the goals themselves, and to variances between goals and actual results, rather than to powers of observation.

Goals may be compatible or incompatible. Goals must be compatible with the supporting processes and systems if we are to have achievement. We noted that any system at work produces results (achieved goals).

Therefore, if a new goal is incompatible with the existing substructure, and no changes are made in the substructure, the old results will continue and the new goals will become empty promises. To expect achievement by simply stating a goal in the context of an incompatible substructure is an idle wish.

Many of these process-system structures are deeply entrenched, and knowledge regarding their resistance to change is advisable before setting objectives. It is perhaps failure to recognize incompatibility and entrenchment that leads many office-seekers to overstate their intentions.

Goals are impossible to reach where the needed processes cannot be defined and/or systems implemented. Goals are impractical where the cost of changing the substructure exceeds the derived benefit.

Goals may be operational or nonoperational. An operational goal lends itself to measurement; a nonoperational goal is purely subjective. An operational goal provides a basis for monitoring progress and achievement, but need not be quantitative in nature. To agree to meet a friend at a certain time and place is an operational goal because you either did or did not meet. (Where operational goals are not quantified we are limited to a yes-no outcome.)

On the other hand, a goal such as improvement of employee morale is nonoperational because what constitutes morale is uncertain in the first place. Many important goals are subjective or nonoperational. For this reason we should seek ways to make them operational rather than abandon them. Improving morale is a case in point. If you ask an executive why he believes morale has improved, he will likely cite an increase in productivity, a decrease in turnover, and other objective indexes to support his claim. If these are, in fact, the means by which morale is measured, then we can formalize these indexes as part of the goal itself.

Indirect measures for subjective goals are termed surrogates.[2] Surrogates for morale might include productivity, turnover, absenteeism, and formal complaints. Only indexes that are capable of objective measurement can be used as surrogates. Also, there must be agreement that certain surrogates will be accepted as the means for operationalizing a goal.

For purposes of measurement, it is necessary to go one step beyond identifying surrogates. They are unlikely to be of equal importance vis-a-

---

[2]A more intensive treatment of the relationship between principals and surrogates is provided by S.I. Hayakawa, *Language in Thought and Action* (2nd ed.; New York: Harcourt, Brace & World, Inc., 1964), Chapter 2, and Yuji, Ijiri, *The Foundations of Accounting Measurement* (Englewood Cliffs, N.J.: Prentice-Hall, Inc., 1967), pp. 1-31.

vis a goal. Hence we must weight them in the order of their perceived importance to a goal:

Productivity	40%
Turnover	30
Absenteeism	20
Formal complaints	10
Morale	*100%*

The above weighting implies that a change in productivity has four times the significance of a change in the number of formal complaints on the issue of morale.

Complex goals such as improvement of morale usually require several surrogates. If only one were needed it should, of course, replace the goal as being a more useful statement of purpose. On the other hand, it is not necessary to exhaust the universe of surrogates. Once we have accounted for 90 percent or more of the goal activity through the weighting of surrogates, the rest can be ignored as being statistically insignificant.[3]

Operational goals provide a number of benefits. In terms of motivation, employees will have a clear picture of what is expected of them and what indexes will be used to measure goal attainment. From a measurement viewpoint, operational goals force us to clarify our objectives, and this in turn facilitates evaluation in that we know the extent to which we have met our objectives.

Processes

A process is *a set of activities pertinent to a goal or result.* Processes can be thought of transformations: food is digested, persons are transported, presidents are elected, raw material is converted into products, and so forth. As noted in these examples, processes move things from one state of nature to another.

Processes are finite or repetitive. Finite (terminal) processes can be represented by a straight line. Examples are the processes of life, production of a product, a college education, or electing a president.

Other processes are repetitive and can be represented by a circle. The function of a repetitive process is to maintain a level of activity. The heart function and circulation are examples in physiology; the weekly payroll is an example in finance. There are processes within processes, and we can

---

[3]This observation is germane to many data collection problems. For example, in obtaining credit information it may not be necessary to exhaust the possible pool of information, but rather to collect data on the most significant surrogates for the complex principals of "character" and "capacity."

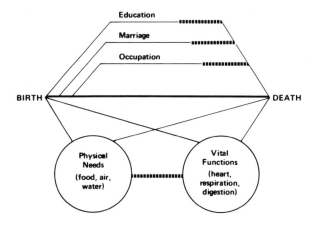

FIGURE 4. Network of Major Life Processes

depict these relationships as networks. A network of the major life processes is illustrated in Figure 4. In all process networks there is one macroprocess. In our example it is the life process beginning with birth and ending with death.

Our observations lead us to believe that all macroprocesses are finite (in the absence of proof of eternity or perpetual motion). Hence, all repetitive processes exist in support of one or more finite processes. The objective of a repetitive process is to maintain a cycle of activity in favor of some larger finite process. There is no aggregation or procession of events in repetitive processes. A repetitive process can be said to succeed or fail on the basis of its ability to maintain a desired level of activity in a larger finite process.

It follows that breakdown in a repetitive process affects some larger finite process. Conversely, ending a finite process also ends its supporting repetitive functions.

Organizations have three major process elements. We refer to this structure as a triprocess complex (see Figure 5, which also illustrates the trisystem complex, discussed in a section that follows).

The macroprocess transforms inputs into outputs. Input-output varies in terms of the function of the organization. Schools transform unskilled persons into skilled ones; manufacturers convert raw materials into products; and accountants produce financial statements out of raw data.

Control ensures that results conform to plans. The purpose of feedback is to monitor transformation activities, report on the state of control,

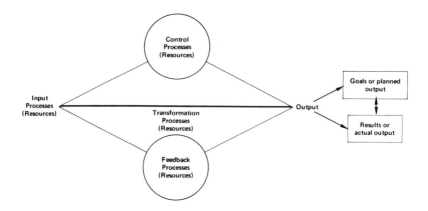

FIGURE 5. The TriProcess (TriSystem) Complex in Organizations

and interpret results. Of course, there are many subprocesses that underlie transformation, control, and feedback.

We shall see that in operating terms triprocess complexes have counterpart trisystem complexes. But let us first consider two problems associated with the management of processes: measurement and formalization.

Processes also pose problems of measurement because there is infinite gradation within processes. For example, we age constantly, not once a year on our birthday. The problem of infinite gradation is resolved through scaling

Scales may be quantitative; for example, we measure time in units such as seconds, minutes, hours, and days. We can measure speed in miles per hour and lifespans in years. Scales may also be qualitative. For example, we may measure the progress in construction of a house in steps: digging for the foundation, erecting the framing, completing the room, and installing the plumbing.

With qualitative scaling persons must be thoroughly familiar with the process in order to monitor progress. For someone knowledgeable in house construction a report to the effect that "we are at the plumbing stage" would be meaningful process information.

For most purposes, however, quantitative scales are necessary. We note that all scales are arbitrary. Why do we measure life in years of age rather than in mental or physiological terms? Why do some measure distance in yards while others use meters? Scales are essentially conventional, and it is difficult to alter long-standing measures as we have noted in the conversion of the British currency and will note in the move toward the metric system in the United States.

Scales can be refined. We now refer to computer speeds in nanoseconds (one-billionth of a second). The refinement of scales conforms to a general rule of economics in that an optimal scale exists at the point where the marginal benefits of refinement exceed marginal costs to the widest extent.

Processes may be formal or informal. We formalize processes through such media as maps, blueprints, flowcharts, descriptions, instructions, guides, organization charts, and manuals. Informal processes are communicated through skill exchanges, work experiences, verbal instructions, and observation. Some fairly complex processes take place without formalization. Persons thoroughly familiar with the process of construction, for example, can build a house without blueprints.

While systems management has made great strides in the past decade, the management of processes is not yet off home base. Many complex processes in organization, not the least being decision processes, are now uncharted. This paucity of formalized processes lies at the root of much mismanagement.

Many informal processes could be formalized if we made the effort. Some processes, which have previously been held to be too complex to formalize, are yielding to advanced techniques such as decision modeling, simulation, and dynamic programming. We can expect greater advances in formalizing processes in the years ahead. Perhaps in time we will even have process specialists. The reason for this prognosis is that our search for efficiency must come to include process factors in addition to systems factors.

Systems

We have defined a system as "a resource network geared to a purposive end"; it is the means by which processes occur. Resources available to systems managers comprise labor, capital, and materials. Combining these resources in meaningful ways enables managers to attain organization goals.

We stated earlier that the triprocess complex has an alter ego in the trisystems complex (Figure 5). We are concerned with the same elements of input, output, feedback, and transformation, but our viewpoint is different. The difference is that we are concerned with the essence of the activity in process terms, but from a systems perspective we are concerned with the mix of resources required to make the process operational. What takes

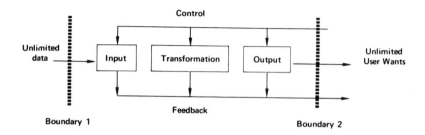

FIGURE 6. An Operating System for Accounting

place in the context of operations defines its processes; how those operations occur defines its systems.

Consider accounting as an operating system. Its purpose is to facilitate the decision-making processes of users. The input is raw data, which are admitted to the accounting system, are transformed, and leave the system in the form of financial reports (Figure 6).

On the one hand, the system faces an environment of unlimited data, while on the other it faces unlimited user wants. No system can cope with these conditions. Accordingly, each system has its limitations as denoted by boundaries 1 and 2. Boundary 1 serves as a screen in that only a portion of the data in the environment is admitted to the system. Boundary 2 serves as a screen in that various users get certain information based on their needs, whether they are entitled to the information, and the constraints (including costs) of providing it. Without boundaries we have no system. The nature of these boundaries also distinguishes one system from another.

The admission of data to the accounting system is not random, that is, we do not take every nth item in a newspaper, for example, and admit it to the system. Rather, well-defined input rules facilitate a rational screening. It follows that there are transformation, control, feedback, and output rules and procedures.

Systems too can be formalized through design and engineering. Many of the devices by which processes are formalized, as described earlier, are used in formalizing systems. Again the difference is substantive—what is being formalized. In the case of processes, we are defining the nature of operations, while in formalizing systems we are designing the utilization of resource elements.

EFFICIENCY

The ultimate objective in management is to reach goals in the most efficient way. Making efficiency judgments requires both process and systems data. For example, the most efficient water delivery project is the one that delivers the greatest quantity of the highest quality water (process data) at the lowest cost and in the least time (systems data).

Process data are qualitative in nature, while systems data are generally expressed in terms of cost or time cost. A process can be said to yield *activity* data, while a system gives us *energy* data. The notion of activity stems from the fact that something is happening in a process, while the concept of energy arises from the fact that resources are being consumed (hence releasing energy) in order to make things happen.

For example, to measure efficiency in operating a delivery truck, we juxtapose an activity scale (mileage or value of deliveries) against an energy scale (operating and maintenance expense). Neither scale alone gives us sufficient data for efficiency judgments. Similarly, the efficiency of a government or any other organization cannot be measured by the amount of its budget or level of its operations (a decrease in the budget is not necessarily an act of efficiency or vice versa). Instead, efficiency is measured in terms of what is accomplished in the light of available resources.

A major characteristic of conventional decision making is an abundance of systems data but a paucity of process data. In an age where qualitative factors are reaching parity with economic concerns, the need to define and measure processes emerges as a major challenge. For this reason, we have sought to make these distinctions clear.

The lack of clarity concerning the use of the terms "process" and "systems" hampers our efforts to manage organizations effectively. These terms bear a close relationship to the goals of an organization. We have expressed this relationship as a goal-process-system or GPS Complex. Goals are defined as objectives, processes as activities, and systems as resource networks. GPS Compelexes can assume different forms, which are the basis for both behavioral and economic considerations.

Examination of the G, P and S elements in more detail indicate that efficiency judgments are only possible in the context of both process and systems data. Our traditional information structures, particularly in accounting, have been rich sources of systems data but are impoverished as to process data. We view this imbalance as a major obstacle to advancing the technology of management. Our hope is that this conceptual treatment will serve at least to highlight a significant problem, and perhaps point to more useful frameworks.

11

Power, Conflict, and Structure In Mental Health Organizations: A General Systems Analysis

THOMAS DOLGOFF

I. INTRODUCTION

"It isn't the things we don't know that get us into trouble: It's the things we know that aren't so."

Many mental health administrators can confirm the wisdom of this adage. They have suffered the consequences of trying to apply to their own settings concepts and principles from industrial, educational, and public administration systems. They are confounded by a bewildering array of theories that view organizations as authority structures, communications linkages, means-ends chains, decision hierarchies, or arenas for interpersonal and intergroup interaction. They look for guidance in many roles — as father or overseer-pacesetter who metes out rewards and punishments, as teacher who instructs and grades, as a political leader who influences and negotiates, as a technical decision-maker, or as a therapist-counselor who manipulates the group and the psychological environment (Sayles 1964; Schein 1965).

The mental health administrator needs a more relevant body of theoretical and empirical knowledge than exists today. Until it emerges, he may find help in the notion that mental health organizations are

FROM: *Administration in Mental Health*, Winter 1972, pp. 12-21.

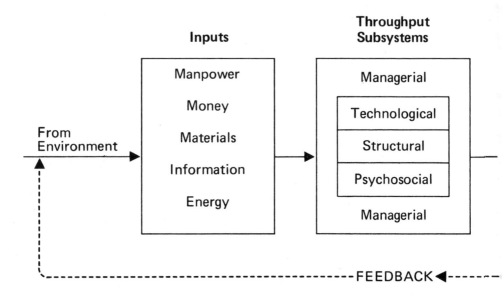

FIGURE 1. Organizations as Socio-Technical Systems

sociotechnical systems (Katz and Kahn 1966; Likert 1961; Rice 1963; Trist et al. 1963). In this view, the organization structures and integrates human activities within and about various technologies. The equipment, tools, facilities, and techniques affect, and are affected by, the social and psychological situation and relationships of persons within and outside the organization.

Figure I summarizes this concept. In the "throughput" or "processing" stage, three subsystems are embedded in a fourth. The technological subsystem is based on the organization's task requirements and the necessary specialized knowledge, skills, equipment, and methods. The psychosocial subsystem includes the expectations, aspirations, and values of individuals and groups; their conflicting and convergent sentiments and beliefs become emotionally charged and determine the organizational atmosphere and climate, since "ideologies create their own morality" (Strauss et al. 1964). The structural subsystem provides the linkage between the technological and psychosocial subsystems. It prescribes the division and coordination of roles and tasks, rules and procedures, the flow of activity and communication, and the patterns of decision and authority. These three subsystems are contained in a fourth, the managerial subsys-

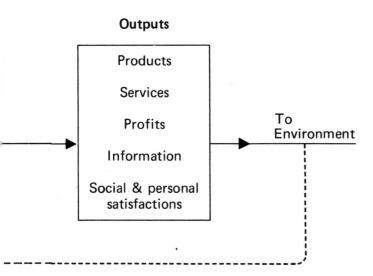

Outputs

Products

Services

Profits

Information

Social & personal
satisfactions

To
Environment

tem; it controls, coordinates, and directs the activities within and between these subsystems, the total organization, and the environment. It is concerned with control, compromise, long-term survival, growth, and efficiency.

In mental health organizations, as in others, the technological, psychosocial, structural, and managerial subsystems are in constant and complex interaction with one another and with the environment in varying degrees of consensus and conflict.

This approach to administration is particularly congenial to mental health professionals because it leans heavily on sociological and psychological concepts and integrates them with concepts derived from industrial settings.

In this paper, the sociotechnical model is illustrated by a study of the interactions of three subsystems in the admission of patients to a psychiatric hospital. (See Figure 2.) It is based on a case presentation in a seminar on mental health administration for first-year psychiatric residents at the Menninger School of Psychiatry. The discussion is limited to staff interactions and to issues of role, power, authority, and conflict that commonly arise in mental health organizations. (The author is deeply indebted to Ann

FIGURE 2.

AN ANALYSIS OF THREE SUBSYSTEMS IN A PSYCHIATRIC HOSPITAL[1]

Subsystem	Input (Resources)	Throughput (Organizational Processes)			Output (Goals)
		Technological Subsystem	Structural Subsystem	Psycho-social Subsystem	
Admissions Officer	Prospective patients. Referring physicians & agencies. Other hospitals, clinics, & social agencies	Diagnostic Skills. Knowledge of suitability & characteristics of other treatment facilities (for referrals). Communication skills with variety of 'publics'.	Roles, procedures, & channels for admission decisions. Mechanisms for processing & disposition of requests for treatment.	Norm of helpfulness. Primary orientation outwards toward referral sources.	Admitted patient who is suitable input for Section Chief. Satisfied referral sources.
Section Chief	Motivated &2 psychologically minded patients likely to benefit from group interaction in a	Diagnosis, treatment, teaching, research, & staff development. Knowledge & application of	Coordination of specialized competencies in interdisciplinary teams	Norms of professional excellence. Desire for self-fulfillment of patients, staff, & trainees.	Healthier patients. Wiser Students. More skillful therapists.

	'therapeutic community'	group dynamics	Staff, patient, & team meetings.	Value of continuity of treatment in timing, place, & personnel. Morale & cohesion in patient-patient, patient-staff, and staff-staff groups.	Healthier patients, wiser students; more skillful & motivated staff.
Medical Director		Planning, organizing, leading, controlling. Integrating diverse goals, values, ideologies, & methods.	Mechanisms & channels for inter-section coordination & communication. Linking technical, maintenance, & adaptive subsystems with each other & the environment.	Control for conflict management & goal attainment. Compromise for maintaining dynamic equilibrium. Long-term survival. Optimum use of resources. Development and maintenance of capacity. Primary orientation towards community for relevance & support.	Satisfied referral sources. Financial solvency. Material & psychological support from geographical, political, & professional communities.
Patients					
Staff					
Trainees					
Funds					
Ideas					
Information					

[1] This chart is a highly simplified schematic representation based on the admission of a patient to one of several sections. It illustrates the relationships presented in more theoretical form in Figure 1.

[2] Patients not meeting these criteria may be rejected by the section, referred to other sections in this hospital, or referred to hospitals or clinics elsewhere.

Appelbaum, M.D., of the Menninger Foundation, Topeka, Kans., for permission to use her unpublished paper upon which this discussion is based.)

No general solutions to administrative dilemmas are offered in this paper. Nor has any attempt been made to provide examples of ways in which the model might be put to practical use. It is felt, however, that the application of general systems theory to mental health administration (both in practice and as a teaching aid) offers the promise of a common language that will enable administrators, professionals, and others to communicate intelligently and productively, and perhaps gain some insight into the reasons behind their conflicts. It may be that such conflicts are inevitable, and, in some ways, beneficial to the organization. This does not lessen the value of the systems approach. A thorough understanding of systems theory and its application to his organization will enable the skilled administrator to heighten the benefits of conflict while reducing its damaging effects.

II. CASE STUDY

A psychiatric hospital recently was decentralized into five semiautonomous sections, each emphasizing a different treatment approach. The admissions officer was responsible for making sure that the following six conditions were met before a new patient was admitted: An available bed; an available doctor; available nursing staff; an available social worker; an available activities therapist; and the "right" patient. The last point is particularly significant because if a patient subsequently turned out to be a poor treatment case, the admissions officer was blamed — implicitly or explicitly — for having given the hospital a "bad" admission.

The admissions officer described how he became more and more cautious about admitting patients and would ask the family or referring physician for detailed information in an effort to make certain that the patient would be a "good" admission.

The following are excerpts from the admission officer's report:

> "With the hospital full and the waiting list lengthening daily, I was bombarded by the human needs of people requesting help. I found that personal satisfaction in this position depended upon being able to respond helpfully. Inability to do so made me feel guilty and frustrated. I saw how in time a person in this position could feel increasingly hostile toward those requesting help that was not available; and how this sense of angry impotence found expression in irritability and

exasperation, which in turn was experienced by patients and referring physicians as rejection, indifference, or contempt. I found myself warding off guilt feelings by giving half-promises to applicants and disappointing them slowly instead of humanely putting an end to their hopes immediately.

Many of these patients might have made good use of the treatment we offer if space had been available. No matter how tactfully or sympathetically the message might be conveyed these applicants felt 'rejected,' could not believe that we really had no room, and sometimes sought other channels for gaining admission.

My compassion for the applicants and my guilt about being unable to help them sometimes made me feel angry with other members of the staff and shift the guilt onto them. I began to see section chiefs, hospital doctors, and the referring physicians as selfish and unfeeling. I thought I noted the same attitude in the staff of the admissions office at various times, and began to realize that this behavior stemmed from the work situation itself rather than from personality characteristics of the individuals involved.

In an attempt to respond to the constantly increasing demands for admission to our hospital I set up weekly meetings where I was in the position of "selling" patients to the section chiefs, who would often say that they could not accept them. I developed an increasingly intense need to get patients into the hospital by one means or another, and I could sometimes find ways to do this. For example, after a section chief told me that he could not admit a certain patient I happened to meet one of this section's doctors in the canteen and was able to convince him to take the case.

Why would I do a thing like that? I did it because I was responsible for admissions without having the authority to bring them about, and because of my frustration in having to refuse help so often while the team had the satisfaction of consummating the admission. This combination of responsibility and ineffectualness led me to identify with my clientele (the referring physicians, their patients and families), perceiving the hospital 'system' as hostile, and seeking ways to circumvent it. All this happened in a situation where I felt strong personal allegiance to the hospital, was in the job for a limited period of time, and was charged with the task of making objective observations!

I believe that the problems I have described would be greatly alleviated if patients were admitted for diagnosis only, with the understanding that the inpatient examination may or may not eventuate in continued treatment here. We would not have to screen applicants so carefully and would be able to admit many more of them. While we might not keep many for long-term treatment, we could give those patients a good diagnostic study and an informed referral for definitive treatment elsewhere. Decisions about admission would be based on objective guidelines and hospital-wide considerations, removed from section loyalties, rivalries and interests. Decisions about continued treatment would be made by the section teams, and could involve transfers of patients between sections in the light of special interests and talents and available beds."

III. ANALYSIS

Role Conflict and Stress. – This report illustrates several types of conflict that are created in organizations, as well as the interaction of organizational, personality, and interpersonal factors in sociotechnical systems. (The concepts of role conflict and stress used in this section are based upon Kahn et al. (1964).)

The admissions officer functions on the boundary between the organization and its environment, as represented by prospective patients and referral sources. Since he is concerned with the input phase of the system, he tends to identify with the attitudes and needs of outsiders and to expouse their interests. The medical director expects him to maintain the census by admitting the optimum number of patients. The section chiefs, however, expect him to produce the "right" patient at the "right" time. (The term "right" is not defined in the same way by all the persons concerned.) The admissions officer is thus subject to "intersender conflict" — incompatible expectations from several persons it is important to please or obey.

He is also exposed to "intraperson conflict" — discrepancies between his internal standards of value and the behavior required of him in the admissions role. This conflict makes it difficult for him to meet "the human needs of people requesting help." It puts him in the uncomfortable position of pressing colleagues to accept patients for reasons of administration and census maintenance rather than for reasons the colleagues regard as more legitimate (i.e., maintaining group cohesion on the ward). He also faces "intrasender conflict" — incompatible expectations from one person. For example, the medical director would like him to keep the census high without creating unnecessary difficulties for the section chiefs or impairing their effectiveness.

Boundaries and Needs

The admissions officer cannot control the flow of demands for admission or the response of the section chiefs to these demands. Yet his own performance depends upon the effective and harmonious interaction of these divergent forces. The misunderstandings that frequently develop across organizational and subsystem boundaries about needs, values, and constraints create many problems for persons in boundary positions. They are blamed by outsiders for shortcomings within their organizations, and by insiders for what outsiders do or fail to do.

The medical director and the section chiefs also are exposed to role conflicts. The medical director must reconcile internal and external demands, maintain standards, job satisfaction, and morale. He must be responsive to the public and protect the hospital's financial viability by maintaining the census. He depends upon the admissions officer to help with these tasks. The section chiefs must provide each patient optimum opportunities for recovery and must protect the conditions which make that possible.

If, instead of the admissions officer, the report had been written by a section chief, for example, he might have described conflicts in terms of giving residents experience in working up patients while ensuring the continuity of treatment by the same therapist. Section chiefs or some of their section members (who do not necessarily agree with one another) may object to the separation of diagnosis and treatment and may thus be exposed to "intraperson conflict" between their values and the demands made upon them.

The common consequences of role conflict, tension, and anxiety, result in cognitive, emotional, and physiological responses that vary in intensity and duration. These stresses often result in withdrawal from, or hostility towards, those creating the conflict, in reduced communication with them, and in derogation of their power. These attitudes influence the perceptions of those to whom they are communicated. They set up a cycle of perceptions and expectations that intensify the underlying problems and often produce self-fulfilling prophecies. Ironically, flexible "other directed" persons (Riesman 1950), such as the admissions officer, are more likely to experience role conflict and stress than rigid "inner directed" persons. "Other directed" persons are more sensitive because of their interaction with others, their need for recognition and approval, and their difficulty in saying "no."

Professional Norms and Organizational Needs

Administrators and professionals in professional organizations often have different views about what work will be done, how it will be done, when, and by whom. The primary function of professionals is to protect the standards for creative activity while administrators must be primarily concerned with the efficient coordination of diverse activities (Dolgoff 1970). The professional says: "I have to be creative." The administrator says: "Creativity is not enough."

These distinctions between professionals and administrators refer to the roles persons play, not to their training, experience, or primary reference group. The admissions officer, in arranging a patient's admission, is an "administrator." But he also functions as a "professional" when he evaluates the clinical indications for admission. When the medical director makes a budgetary decision, he is an "administrator." When an administrator teaches administration, he assumes a "professional" teaching role. Regardless of such role reversals, however, persons functioning as administrators usually administer "means" rather than "ends," and, as a result, are often accused of permitting techniques to triumph over purpose.

Administrators in organizations employing professionals must often assert the right to select the organization's customers, clients, patients, or research problems. Professional schools emphasize that the professional must have a free choice in such matters. The admissions officer's report reveals how the organization's screening processes may thus be a source of conflict (Abrahamson 1967).

The problems of patient flow in a decentralized hospital illustrate organizational stresses that reflect the more general dilemmas of differentiation and integration, creativity and compliance, freedom and order (Dale 1969). Organizational units with different task requirements, such as the admissions office and the clinical sections, tend to acquire different characteristics, norms, and values, consistent with their tasks.

What is functional for one subsystem may be dysfunctional for other subsystems or the organization as a whole. While a particular section may prefer empty beds to the admission of a patient for whom their treatment program is not designed, the hospital as a whole must maintain an adequate census to remain financially solvent. In such a case, the section chief and admissions officer may accuse each other of displacing the organization's goals.

Power, Authority, and Responsibility

The admissions officer is expected to maintain the census by regulating the flow of patients into the hospital. He complains that he is "responsible for admissions without the authority to bring them about." Power is necessary when a decision must be made and consensus cannot be reached — a common situation in psychiatric organizations where there are incompatible goals, needs, norms, and task requirements among individuals and formal and informal groups (Dolgoff 1970; Hersch 1968).

Lacking formal power over "insiders" as well as "outsiders," the admissions officer has to rely heavily on persuasion, and the affective bonds of trust, respect, and sympathy. These bonds are difficult to maintain when the parties whose interests he must reconcile, such as referring doctors and section chiefs, have divergent interests and role pressures (Kahn et al. 1964).

Professionals tend to resist the authority of hierarchical supervisors because their norms prescribe that they are the sole judge of the validity of their own decisions. Furthermore, professionals in administrative roles requiring the exercise of power are often apologetic and embarrassed about exercising that power — partly because of the conflict with their professional norms, and often because of their failure to distinguish between legitimate and necessary power (authority) and its arbitrary use (authoritarianism) (Dolgoff 1970; Abrahamson 1967).

The section chiefs, of course, could make the same complaint about the admissions officer that he makes about them. They are responsible for the treatment of the patients on their sections, but are under administrative pressure to accept patients without due regard for the type of patients, the timing of their admission, or their compatibility with other patients or with staff capabilities and needs. They could compare their plight with that of a manufacturer who is unable to control the amount or quality of the raw materials, but is responsible for the quality of the manufactured product.

Displacement of Goals

An organization is said to displace its goals when it substitutes for its legitimate goals some other goals for which it was not created and for which resources were not allocated. Goals may be displaced because of vested interests of leaders and members and fixation on internal problems. In this case report, the goals of subsystems displaced the broader goals of the hospital, or vice versa, depending on who is making the judgment — the admissions officer or the section chief. The admissions officer could say that the overriding goals of financial solvency, service responsibilities to the local community, and training needs for the larger community were all being jeopardized by the narrow parochialism of the section chiefs. The section chiefs could counter that the admissions officer was sacrificing professional values and the needs of patients to crass monetary considerations and a good public relations image.

The Informal Organization

When a section chief refuses to accept a certain patient, the admissions officer finds a way to reverse his decision by circumventing the formal structure. He meets one of the section's doctors in the canteen and induces him to accept the patient. This incident illustrates the importance of the informal organization — small groups or societies that often do not coincide with the groupings within the formal organization. They are governed by the "logic of sentiments" rather than by the formal organization's "logic of efficiency." They provide opportunities for social interaction, feelings of status, self-esteem, self-expression, and group acceptance, and enable the organization to carry out the group's "expressive"needs (Parsons 1964). The canteen incident also illustrates how informal arrangements can be more flexible and spontaneous than formal ones, and can protect the organization from damage that may result from literal obedience to formal roles, policies, and regulations (Davis 1957; Mayo 1954; Roethlisberger 1951).

Boundary Controls and Ego Psychology

A.K. Rice (1969) suggests that the individual and the group may be seen as open systems as well as subsystems within an organization. This case illustrates his theory that each transaction involving individuals or groups challenges the integrity of the boundaries across which it takes place, as well as the legitimacy of authority in boundary regulation and control.

The interaction between the admissions office and the sections illustrates how each organization unit has its own primary and secondary tasks, its own constraints, and its own boundaries and boundary control functions. Each system attempts to integrate task needs and constraints with the roles, norms, and emotional requirements of individuals and groups. In each system, the administrator is analogous to the ego as it checks and measures intakes, controls conversion processes, and inspects outputs. These are the classical functions of the administrator (planning, organizing, directing, coordinating, and budgeting).

Organizational ineffectiveness, therefore, can be likened to psychopathology in an individual in that both are due to the breakdown of the control function: ego in the individual and management in the organization (Menninger 1963).

IV. SUMMARY

This paper uses the case approach in analyzing mental health administration. An objective of the systems analysis employed here is to help students move back and forth between the world of the theorist and the world of the practitioner, and to experience as well as conceptualize the interrelationships of organizational functions and structures, and the complexity and diversity of goals, norms, values, incentives, and power strategies in mental health agencies.

References

Abrahamson, Mark. 1967. *The Professional in the Organization.* Chicago: Rand-McNally.

Dale, Ernest. 1969.*Management Theory and Practice.*New York: McGraw-Hill.

Dolgoff, Thomas. 1970. The organization, the administrator and the mental health professional. *Hospital & Community Psychiatry,*21: 45-52.

Davis, Keith. 1957. *Human Relations in Business.*New York: McGraw-Hill.

Hersch, Charles. 1968. The discontent explosion in mental health. *American Psychologist,* 23: 497-506.

Kahn, Robert L., et al. 1964. *Organizational Stress: Studies in Role Conflict and Ambiguity.* New York: John Wiley & Sons.

Katz, Daniel, and Kahn, Robert L. 1966. *The Social Psychology of Organizations.* New York: John Wiley & Sons.

Likert, Rensis. 1961. *New Patterns of Management.* New York: McGraw-Hill.

Mayo, Elton. 1954. *The Social Problems of an Industrial Civilization.* Boston: Harvard University Graduate School of Business.

Menninger, Karl, et al. 1963. *The Vital Balance.* New York: Viking Press.

Parsons, Talcott. 1964. *The Social System.* New York: Free Press.

Rice, A. K. 1963. *The Enterprise and Its Environment.* London: Tavistock.

Rice, A. K. 1969. Individual, group and intergroup processes.*Human Relations,* 6: 565-584.

Riesman, David. 1950. *The Lonely Crowd: A Study of the Changing American Character.* New Haven: Yale University Press.

Roethlisberger, Fritz J. 1951. *Management and Morale.* Cambridge: Harvard University Press.

Sayles, Leonard R. 1964. *Managerial Behavior.* New York: McGraw-Hill.

Schein, Edgar H. 1965. *Organizational Psychology.* Englewood Cliffs, N.J.: Prentice Hall.

Strauss, Anselm L. et al. 1964. *Psychiatric Ideologies and Institutions.* New York: Free Press.

Trist, Eric L., et al. 1963. *Organizational Choice.* London: Tavistock.

Bibliography

Belknap, Ivan. *Human Problems in a State Mental Hospital.* New York: McGraw-Hill, 1956.

Bertalanffy, Ludwig von. *General System Theory, Foundations, Development, Applications.* New York: G. Braziller, 1968.

Buckley, Walter. *Sociology and Modern System Theory.* Englewood Cliffs, N.J.: Prentice Hall, 1967.

Buckley, Walter. *Modern System Research for the Behavioral Scientist: A Source Book.* Chicago: Aldine, 1968.

Etzioni, Amitai. *Modern Organizations*. Englewood Cliffs, N.J.: Prentice Hall, 1964.

Goffman, Erving. *Asylums*. Garden City, N.Y.: Doubleday, Anchor Books, 1961.

Gray, William, et al., eds. *General Systems Theory and Psychiatry*. Boston: Little, Brown & Co., 1969.

Herzberg, Frederick. *Work and the Nature of Man*. New York: World Publishing Co., 1966.

Katz, Daniel, and Kahn, Robert L. *The Social Psychology of Organizations*. New York: John Wiley & Sons, 1966.

Lawrence, Paul R., and Lorsch, Jay W. *Developing Organizations: Diagnosis and Action*. Reading, Mass.: Addison-Wesley, 1969.

Menzies, Isabel E.P. A case study in the functioning of social systems as a defense against anxiety. *Human Relations*, 13: 95-121, May 1960.

Miller, James G., Toward a general theory for the behavioral sciences. *American Psychologist*, 10: 513-531, Sept. 1955.

Rosenthal, Robert, and Jacobson, Lenore. *Pygmalion in the Classroom; Teacher Expectation and Pupils' Intellectual Development*. New York: Holt, Rinehart & Winston, 1968.

Ullman, Leonard P. *Institution and Outcome: A Comparative Study of Psychiatric Hospitals*. Oxford, N.Y.: Pergamon Press, 1967.

12

Systems Theory, Organizations, and Management

WARREN B. BROWN

In recent years it has been easy to note a sharp upswing in the use of the term *systems*; examples are systems theory, systems analysis, managerial systems, urban systems, and transportation systems. Assuming that this usage reflects something more than a fad, is it reasonable to ask what is this concept that has generated such widespread usage.

The emphasis in this article will be on exploring with the reader the meaning and usefulness of the systems concept, with special emphasis on the relationship between systems theory and problems dealing with organization and management. One approach will be to examine the reasons for its increasingly pervasive usage; another will be to look at its limitations in order to keep the discussion in perspective. Consideration of the following topics will include, as needed, the development of some of the vocabulary appropriate to this field.

General systems theory.
Systems concepts and characteristics.
The organization as an open system.
The organization and the task environment.
Systems analysis and managerial decision-making.
Limitations.

FROM: *Oregon Business Review*, June 1970, pp. 1-6.

GENERAL SYSTEMS THEORY

What is a system? Although any one definition is somewhat arbitrary, most definitions have in common some elements that can be applied to all types of systems. Here the term *system* will refer simply to a group or complex of parts such as people or machines interrelated in their actions toward some goal(s). The generality of this concept is the underlying reason that it has been found useful as a framework for the exploration of all kinds of phenomena: physical, biological, social, economic, etc.

Too much generality, however, does not satisfy the demand for the understanding of detailed phenomena; hence, next comes consideration of subsystems and levels of analysis. Boulding provides the following classification of system levels:

1. The static structure: the general anatomy or framework of a system.
2. The simple dynamic system: a system analogous to a clockwork, with necessary, predetermined motions.
3. The cybernetic system: a system able to regulate itself so as to maintain a position of equilibrium, such as a thermostat.
4. The open system: a self-maintaining system capable of internal change, growth, and reproduction. Living systems begin at this level.
5. The genetic-societal system: this level is characterized by cells, cell differentiation, and plant life.
6. The animal system: characterized by mobility and goal-directed behavior.
7. Human systems: these include self-awareness and the ability to handle symbols, languages, and abstract ideas.
8. Social systems: human organizations with value systems, histories, and the whole range of human interactions.
9. Transcendental systems: ultimate values, absolutes, religious systems—these also are interpreted as exhibiting systematic structure. [3]

If universals can be found which are valid at more than one of these levels, they greatly simplify the quest for knowledge. The study of physical systems (dealing at the first three levels) has led to several scientific laws concerning system behavior at these levels, for example in physics. Similarly, studies at the next three levels, dealing with biological and related systems, have also led to general concepts which seem to be valid for more than one level. In studies of organization and administration, primarily at levels seven and eight in the above classification, there is a search for an empirical and conceptual base of this integrating nature.

The systems approach can thus provide a macroview from which one may study a wide variety of systems. Such studies have been a healthy contrast and supplement to the many studies along traditional subject-matter lines within organizations.

There is a danger in this approach which must quickly be mentioned, however. In the study of systems, it becomes tempting to analyze a relatively simple, lower level system and then try to generalize from the underlying characteristics of that analysis to higher level, and more complex, systems. These analogies have been constructed to link many differing phenomena: an example is the analogy between feedback control models in electronic circuitry and information flow on the one hand and control concepts in human organizations on the other.

The difficulties of demonstrating the validity of such an analogy often are sizable; for the two systems to be analogous, their key elements must be virtually isomorphic (exhibiting a one-to-one relationship), and the operational relationships among the elements of the systems must be implicitly identical. In short, knowledge of one kind of phenomenon may seem satisfying and fairly complete, but care must be taken in extrapolating that knowledge to another level of analysis. Understanding the social system of a bee hive may not help much with understanding urban social systems!

Despite difficulties of extrapolation and abstractness, systems theory has helped synthesize and integrate the recent explosion of knowledge in several areas in the physical, biological, and social sciences. By forcing its users to define system elements and to study their interrelationships and the interaction between them and their environment, systems theory provides a valuable framework for understanding many kinds of social, organizational, and administrative phenomena.

SYSTEMS CONCEPTS AND CHARACTERISTICS[1]

One basic characteristic of a system is that it is either open or closed. Closed systems have "information-tight" controls on their activities (they are self-contained and isolated from their environment) and are exemplified by mechanical systems capable of maintaining a position of equilibrium via a feedback control mechanism. Common examples are the Watts governor for the control of engine speeds and the household thermostat for temperature. As illustrated in Figure 1, the typical procedure involves a constant monitoring of the system output; a comparison of the output values with the preset standards; evaluation of any discrepancies; and a flow of information concerning the degree of deviation back to the other elements in the system structure so that the procedures may be changed as necessary.

For fully mechanistic systems, with only deterministic elements in the

---

[1]Some of the discussion of this topic is from the author's article, "Systems, Boundaries, and Information Flow" [5].

structure and with all control procedures consisting of direct coupling and feedback mechanisms, there is complete automation. Introducing human factors into systems of course creates more variability. Note that information-tight systems may be open in terms of other flows, such as materials and energy, through input-output processes.

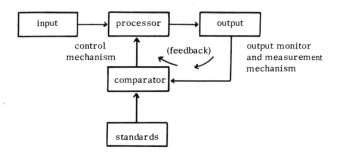

FIGURE 1. A Closed-Loop System with Feedback

By contrast, an open system is affected by its environment; it does not have the information-tight control units characteristic of closed systems. Instead, the relations among the elements of the system, and between the system and its environment, are often unknown, and the precise causes of system changes may be a mystery. Examples are an individual's behavior, a nation's economy, and a rocket system where there is no further control once the rocket has been fired. (Figure 2 illustrates an example of an open system.)

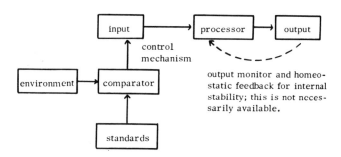

FIGURE 2. An Open System

Even in the case where one does not have complete knowledge or control of the internal workings of a system, it may still be possible to make many inferences about the interrelationships of the system elements. The technique used is called the "Black Box" approach,[2] wherein the system analyst tries to deduce the nature of the internal workings by manipulating the inputs to the system and observing the consequent outputs. For large, complex systems this approach obviously presents many practical difficulties.

Open systems are capable of bringing in from their environment resources by which they can modify their own internal flows, procedures, and structure. In this way they prevent the entropic process, which is well known in physical and biological systems: if there are no counteracting forces, entropy (a measure of the unavailable energy in a system) increases toward a maximum, and the system elements become more randomized and less differentiated. The result of the entropic process is that the system runs down and achieves equilibrium at the most probable distribution of the elements.

This phenomenon can be counteracted by open systems obtaining from their environment more energy and resources than they expend in their operations. They can store resources for possible future crises and otherwise utilize these additional resources for deliberate system changes, such as adaptation and growth which are in accord with system goals.

Open systems also have the characteristics of striving to maintain a dynamic balance (homeostasis). As the environment changes, an open system will monitor these changes and try to adapt itself in keeping with its character and goals. This leads over time to the notion of an open system, such as a human organization, having a dynamic equilibrium rather than a static one.

Another key aspect of describing a system is to separate those elements which belong to the system (or subsystem, as the case may be) from the elements in its environment. The separation is rarely absolute, i.e., some of the elements in the system typically will interact with those in the system environment. For human organizations, the amount of interaction can be thought of in terms of the permeability of the organization's boundaries. This refers to the flow of both people and information across the boundary. The degree of permeability will affect the adaptation of the organization to its environment.

Some organization boundaries are easily penetrated; examples are those of voluntary civic organizations and of political groups [10, pp. 59-62,

---

[2]For a good discussion of this concept, see S. Beer, *Cybernetics* and Management [1, chap. 6].

122-124]. Under such conditions, persons can enter or leave the organization largely at their own will. The other extreme occurs when a person has no choice about his membership in an organization, as when a citizen is drafted by a society into its army. Business firms tend to lie between these extremes, with an individual's hiring and firing often occurring in a semi-voluntary manner due to practical complications such as union restrictions, seniority rights, and so on.

Because people and information coming into an organization will bring knowledge and values from the external environment, the relative permeability of an organization's boundaries affects the degree to which the organization's members are exposed to such influences. If the boundaries effect a tight screening of both information and individuals, so that only those people and pieces of information which reinforce the current internal values are allowed in, then the organization may facilitate internal agreement among its members. However, at the same time it may lose its position in its environment, such as when a firm gets into a rut with its technology and product line. Too loose a screening, on the other hand, may permit disruptive forces to affect adversely the organization's progress toward its goals. An alert management often can select the degree of boundary permeability which seems to fit best the needs of the organization.

A related term often used in systems studies is *interface*, which refers to the points of contact between two subsystems, such as the interface between the marketing and manufacturing divisions in a business firm. Interface problems are essentially ones of communication and coordination among the areas (or groups of people) defined as subsystems.

Subsystems lead to the concept of a hierarchy of systems (such as was mentioned above in describing a general classification of system levels). Generally speaking, all systems can be defined so that each one is considered one part of a larger system and yet in turn is composed of subsystems. Hierarchies appear to be a universal aspect of complex systems; they evolve or are planned in order to coordinate activities and allow for specialization among the subsystem elements. In human organizations, hierarchies are based first on small work groups, then on departments, divisions, companies, conglomerates, and economies. The concept allows for successively inclusive system levels, each of which may be studied either as a separate system or as a subpart of a broader system.

THE ORGANIZATION AS AN OPEN SYSTEM

To understand better the impact of systems thinking on organization analysis, a brief look at some earlier contributions will be helpful.[3] A common starting point is Weber's analysis of bureaucracy, which views the organization as a system of highly formalized roles, structured along superior-subordinate relationships, with the purpose of utilizing the principle of division of labor in order to achieve a high degree of efficiency regarding goal attainment. The operations are maintained through close coordination and control via an elaboration of rules and regulations. The emphasis is on building a smooth-working and efficient organization.

The "scientific management" approach has much the same spirit but more of an industrial engineering flavor. Particularly in the context of manufacturing organizations, this management style emphasized the application of scientific techniques to study and improve even the most minute work methods in all jobs, leading, for example, to standardized techniques in time and motion study. Efficiency in a rather mechanical sense was the main thrust, and many engineering-oriented managers were quick to utilize some of the production methods which evolved.

Again with a focus on organizational rationality, there were some parallel efforts to discover common, underlying principles of management which would serve as guidelines for managers of virtually all types of organizations. These efforts, often labelled the "administrative management school," were very much concerned with basic problems of line and staff relationships, managerial span-of-control, the organizational chain-of-command, etc. The attempt to find standard solutions to these problems, i.e., principles with universal applicability, was unsuccessful, however, as the early statements were so ambiguous, with undefined terms, that they could not be subjected to empirical testing, and indeed were rather confusing to the thoughtful manager.

Partly as a reaction to these earlier emphases on rationality, the human relations studies brought out the importance of human motivation and social forces in the workings of any organization. The human being and the work group became focal points for large numbers of behaviorally oriented studies, with psychologists and social psychologists finding the business firm a rich laboratory for their explorations in studying human behavior.

However, all of these approaches are essentially closed system frameworks; the focus is on internal organizational relationships and economic efficiency, with little if any attention paid to the organization-environment relationship. Yet the organization fits the model of an open system quite well: it receives inputs from the environment, transforms them, and supplies outputs to the environment, the whole pattern representing in the abstract the same cycle as one finds in many biological systems. For a business firm, the inputs are factors like materials, capital,

---

[3]A nice discussion of historical thought leading up to modern theory is in N. P. Mouzelis, *Organization and Bureaucracy* [11].

land, labor, and information. These are combined and transformed into the goods and services which are the firm's output. Through the market mechanism and other intra-organizational relationships, these outputs then provide the resources which enable the firm to remain viable in its environment and to maintain the support of its members.

This is, of course, a rather simple description of a business firm. Although the analogy between the general concept of an open system and a business enterprise may seem intuitively acceptable, the question must be asked: What does this concept provide that the earlier ones mentioned above did not The answer lies in the variables and the interactions that must be examined in order to understand and describe a system. For example, three basic system characteristics relevant to organizations are:

1. Flows: of information, materials, money, etc.;
2. Structure: referring to physical and geographic aspects and to organizational design; and
3. Procedures: the preplanned activities which affect the flows and structure.

Far more than previous concepts, the systems approach allows one to represent adequately the complexity of interrelationships which typify the modern organization, and to include in the analysis the dynamic forces for change as well as those control mechanisms which help maintain stability. The complex organization is thus viewed as a set of interdependent parts, each of which receives some resources from the organization and contributes something in return, with the broader organization always linked to and interdependent with its environment.

THE ORGANIZATION AND THE TASK ENVIRONMENT[4]

With the systems approach demanding a closer look at the organization-environment interaction, it is natural that in recent years there have been some fresh attempts to analyze this area. Thompson [13, p. 26] proposes the concept of organizational domain, focusing on 1) the range of products, 2) the population served, and 3) the services rendered. The domain thus identifies the areas of potential dependency for the organization in terms of separable units in the environment.

The environment refers broadly to "everything else." For simplification, Thompson refers to Dill's study [7] for the narrower concept of task

---

[4]For more details concerning this area, including a study applying these concepts to professional organizations, see the author's article, "The Impact of a Dynamic Task Environment" [6].

environment, i.e., those parts of the environment which are "relevant or potentially relevant to goal setting and goal attainment." In that study of two Norwegian firms [7, pp. 409-443], Dill described their task environments in terms of four factors: 1) customers, including distributors and users, 2) suppliers of materials, labor capital, etc. 3) competitors for both markets and resources, and 4) regulatory groups both public and private.

In further analysis, Thompson [13 p. 72] postulates that task environments also are characterized by two basic dimensions: homogeneous-heterogeneous and stable-dynamic. Examining in particular the boundary-spanning units of an organization, he shows how these would be functionally differentiated to correspond to the organization's task environment. As a firm's environment becomes more heterogeneous, it brings greater constraints to the organization, and it demands a greater variety of functional skills and divisions in response. Also, as the environment becomes more dynamic, it forces more contingencies on the organization. With both a heterogeneous and a dynamic task environment, one would expect the boundary units to be functionally differentiated, corresponding to the relevant factors in the task environment, with each operating as a decentralized unit in order to monitor and respond to changes in its sector.

Thus the task environment concept refers to those aspects of an organization's environment which affect its goal setting and the definition of its domain. These factors introduce and define the dependence of the organization; this in turn generates constraints and contingencies for it. We expect that rationally acting organizations will attempt to minimize their dependency and will strive to do that by utilizing two basic strategies: a competitive strategy or a cooperative strategy. Cooperation involves several distinct degrees of commitment of exchange with other organizations in the task environment: a) contracting, primarily referring to formal commitments for the exchange of performances in the future; b) co-opting, defined by Selznick [12] to mean the absorption of new elements into an organization's policy-determining structure in order to avert threats to its stability or existence; and c) coalescing, referring to a joint venture with one or more organizations in the environment. All of these variations can be found easily by examining modern business practice.

SYSTEMS ANALYSIS AND MANAGERIAL DECISION-MAKING

As well as providing a framework for examining large-scale organizational behavior, the systems approach also has been used increasingly to study managerial decision-making, especially at the policy level. In essence, this approach refers to a way of looking at policy problems to enable the decision-maker to come to better decisions than through other techniques. The systems approach does not necessarily use sophisticated mathematical techniques.[5] It does emphasize a blending of judgment and experience with formal analysis (often a difficult accomplishment in practice) and can be characterized in several ways, some of which relate to the discussion above of large-scale system characteristics.[6]

There is an emphasis on defining the problems (or asking the "right" questions) so that the underlying structure regarding the decision to be made is clearly recognized. This may permit the manager to compare various alternative decisions and improve his understanding of the connections between the organization's goals and the decision systems used to achieve them. However, in most private and public policy areas, e.g., defense or welfare, the number of relevant variables is so large and their interrelationships are so complex that full understanding of the structure behind the decision is exceedingly difficult, and other means must be sought.

The way around the difficulty often is to use proximate goals as a substitute for those which are virtually unmeasurable. As an example, in many business firms the variables of earnings, dividends, and market share may become approximate goals for the more general and vague concept of profit.

Another characteristic is that uncertainities are dealt with in a forthright and explicit manner. Typically, the uncertainties in a problem are transformed into statements of mathematical probability and then are utilized as rationally as the formulations allow. This emphasis on clarity even in the areas where uncertainties prevail is a hallmark of the systems approach and often makes it qualitatively different from other policy treatments.

An additional barrier to clarity arises from the fact that policy problems are generally characterized as a multiobjective situation.[7] Unfortunately for purposes of analysis, these objectives often seem unrelated, and one cannot combine them into a single comprehensive goal, nicely measur-

---

[5]"Operations research" is a related term that has much in common with systems analysis; the differences are primarily a matter of emphasis. In usual usage, operations research focuses on operational level problems, especially those that are amenable to detailed analysis and quantification with a resulting emphasis on mathematical models, whereas systems analysis examines the more abstract and less well-structured policy problems.

[6]For further discussion of this area, especially as related to military strategy, see C. J. Hitch and R. McKean, *The Economics of Defense in the Nuclear Age* [8], and T. C. Whitehead, "Uses and Limitations of Systems Analysis" [14].

[7]A quite comprehensive treatment of the multiobjective decision problem is in E. Johnsen, *Studies in Multiobjective Decision Models* [9].

able along only one dimension. To get at an understanding and analysis of this type of situation, the problem must be factored into a series of subproblems. As Whitehead puts it:

> By identifying cohesive problem areas whose internal relationships can be fairly well understood and which have relatively few links to other problem areas, we can reduce the intellectual capacity required to deal with the larger problem. In effect, each subproblem is solved independently, and the solutions then are combined to produce the total solution. Combining the solutions will, of course, necessitate going back and adjusting the original solutions to account for the interactions among the subproblem areas, but several repetitions of this process are feasible while simultaneous treatment of all the relationships usually is not. The effect of such an approach is the use of whatever models are appropriate for each individual subproblem. And the definition of the subarenas will depend on the particular characteristics of the decision to be made at a given time. The result is an approach to analysis that uses a number of *ad hoc* models to represent the aspects of the alternatives and the environment that are relevant to the particular decision to be made. [14, p.51]

Involved in this factoring process are the use of judgment and the distinction between value judgments and judgments regarding questions of fact, though the two cannot always be separated. In many treatments of decision analysis, value judgments are treated as a given factor, to be taken into account along with factual aspects when the analysis is made. By contrast, systems analysis treats value judgments as variables in the problem and, by virtue of the analysis and improved information, tries to give the decision-maker better insights as to what the implications of his value judgments are. It is possible that with a better understanding of the structure of a problem, some refinement of the original value judgments may be very reasonable.

LIMITATIONS

The systems approach to organizational and managerial problems has not been without criticism [see, for example, 4]. As more persons have become enthusiastic about systems analysis, almost inevitably some exaggerations and misunderstandings have arisen. Here are a few of the main criticisms:

1. The concern for the "totality" of a system often is not reduced to meaningful specifics for problem analysis, but remains only as a very general statement. To speak of "all the elements" of a business organization may serve only to confuse attempts at clarity for problem definition. It becomes important to distinguish among levels of abstraction and analysis and to separate key variables

from less important ones—hence the concern for understanding a problem's structure.

2. Factoring the comprehensive policy problems into more specific, individual subproblems almost inevitably leads to the phenomenon of suboptimization. At times this cannot be avoided; when problem complexity simply overwhelms one's ability to deal with it in a uniform and comprehensive fashion, then one is forced to factor a large problem into smaller ones, striving to structure the factoring in such a manner that the local, individual optimizations will produce a total result not greatly at variance from a theoretical, global optimum.

3. The evolution of many quantitative tools, such as linear programming and computer simulation techniques, as aids in systems analysis has sometimes led to an overemphasis on problems which are quantifiable and especially those which lend themselves to analysis by well-established methods. This may dangerously reduce the importance of factors and problems which are ill structured or contain difficulties of measurement. The policy problems in large organizations remain rather qualitative, however, and demand broad vision rather than tool-orientation.

4. A further criticism relates to the apparent lack of focus on people themselves. As systems analysts become increasingly concerned with computer hardware, system procedures, functional analyses, and heuristic programs, they decreasingly focus on the role of human beings in these newly designed man-machine systems. The critics say that this is just the "scientific management" philosophy in new garb, but with the same basic problems caused by a treatment of human and social factors as manipulable, mechanical elements in the system [2]. This criticism is probably the most far-reaching of the group.

CONCLUSION

The systems approach has many aspects, as is evident even in this short discussion. It has extended several traditional views of organizations, and has brought into focus the "openness" of human organizations and their interrelationships with their environments.

The systems approach has also furthered a kind of problem analysis, especially at the policy level, which has stimulated much new thinking in this area. Though not without criticism, systems analysts have been able to help clarify the conceptual frameworks for decisions, construct alternative plans of action, evaluate the impact of value factors as well as factual considerations, and generally aid in making policy problems explicit. There seems little doubt that the systems approach to organizational and managerial issues will be used increasingly in our complex world.

References

1. S. Beer, *Cybernetics and Management*. N.Y.: Wiley, 1959.
2. R. Boguslaw, *The New Utopians*. Englewood Cliffs, N.J.: Prentice-Hall, 1965.
3. K. E. Boulding, "General Systems Theory: The Skeleton of Science," *Management Science*, Apr. 1956.
4. W. M. A. Brooker, "The Total Systems Myth," *Systems and Procedures Journal*, July-Aug. 1965.
5. Warren B. Brown, "Systems, Boundaries, and Information Flow," *Academy of Management Journal*, Dec. 1966.
6. ———, "The Impact of a Dynamic Task Environment," *Academy of Management Journal*, June 1969.
7. W. R. Dill, "Environment as an Influence on Managerial Autonomy," *Administrative Science Quarterly*, vol. 2, 1958.
8. C. J. Hitch and R. McKean, *The Economics of Defense in the Nuclear Age*. Cambridge: Harvard University Press, 1960.
9. E. Johnsen, *Studies in Multiobjective Decision Models*. N.Y. Barnes and Noble, 1969.

What are your
Organization's Objectives?
A General-Systems Approach to Planning

BERTRAM M. GROSS

There is nothing that managers and management theorists are more solidly agreed on than the vital role of objectives in the managing of organizations. The daily life of executives is full of such exhortations as:

'Let's plan where we want to go . . .'
'You'd better clarify your goals . . .'
'Get those fellows down (or up) there to understand what our (or their) purposes really are . . .'

Formal definitions of management invariably give central emphasis to the formulation or attainment of objectives. Peter Drucker's (1954) idea of 'managing by objectives' gave expression to a rising current in administrative theory. Any serious discussion of planning, whether by business enterprises or government agencies, deals with the objectives of an organization.

Yet there is nothing better calculated to embarrass the average executive than the direct query: 'Just what are your organization's objectives?' The typical reply is incomplete or tortured, given with a feeling of

FROM: *Human Relations*, Vol. 18, August 1965, pp. 195-215.

obvious discomfort. The more skilfull response is apt to be a glib evasion or a glittering generality.

To some extent, of course, objectives cannot be openly stated. Confidential objectives cannot be revealed to outsiders. Tacit objectives may not bear discussion among insiders. The art of bluff and deception with respect to goals is part of the art of administration.

But the biggest reason for embarrassment is the lack of a well-developed language of organizational purposefulness. Such a language may best be supplied by a general-systems model that provides the framework for 'general-systems accounting', or 'managerial accounting' in the sense of a truly generalist approach to all major dimensions of an organization. It is now possible to set forth—even if only in suggestive form—a general-systems model that provides the basis for clearly formulating the performance and structural objectives of any organization.

Let us now deal with these points separately—and conclude with some realistic observations on the strategy of planning.

THE NEED FOR A LANGUAGE OF PURPOSEFULNESS

Many managers are still too much the prisoners of outworn, single-purpose models erected by defunct economists, engineers, and public administration experts. Although they know better, they are apt to pay verbal obeisance to some single purpose: profitability in the case of the business executive, efficiency in the case of the public executive.

If profitability is not the sole objective of a business—and even the more tradition-ridden economists will usually accept other objectives in the form of constraints or instrumental purposes—just what are these other types? If efficiency is not the only objective of a government agency—and most political scientists will maintain that it cannot be—what are the other categories? No adequate answers to these questions are provided by the traditional approaches to economics, business administration, or public administration. Most treatises on planning—for which purpose formulation is indispensable—catalogue purposes by such abstract and non-substantive categories as short-range and long-range, instrumental and strategic (or ultimate), general and specific. One book on planning sets forth thirteen dimensions without mentioning anything so mundane as profitability or efficiency (LeBreton & Henning, 1961). Indeed, in his initial writings on management by objectives, Drucker never came to grips with the great multiplicity of business objectives. In his more recent work Drucker (1964) deals with objectives in terms of three 'result areas': product, distribution channels, and markets. But this hardly goes far enough to illuminate the complexities of purpose multiplicity.

Thus far, the most systematic approach to organizational purposes is provided by budget experts and accountants. A budget projection is a model that helps to specify the financial aspects of future performance. A balance sheet is a model that helps to specify objectives for future structure of assets and liabilities. Yet financial analysis—even when dignified by the misleading label 'managerial accounting'—deals only with a narrow slice of real-life activities. Although it provides a way of reflecting many objectives, it cannot by itself deal with the substantive activities underlying monetary data. Indeed, concentration upon budgets has led many organizations to neglect technological and other problems that cannot be expressed in budgetary terms. Overconcentration on the enlargement of balance-sheet assets has led many companies to a dangerous neglect of human and organizational assets.

The great value of financial analysis is to provide a doorway through which one can enter the whole complex domain of organizational objectives. To explore this domain, however, one needs a model capable of dealing more fully with the multiple dimensions of an organization's performance and structure. To facilitate the development of purposefulness in each of an organization's subordinate units, the model should also be applicable to internal units. To help executives to deal with the complexities of their environment, it should also be applicable to external competitors or controllers.

THE GENERAL-SYSTEMS APPROACH

As a result of the emerging work in systems analysis, it is now possible to meet these needs by developing a 'general-systems model' of an organization. A general-systems model is one that brings together in an ordered fashion information on all dimensions of an organization. It integrates concepts from all relevant disciplines. It can help to expand financial planning to full-bodied planning in as many dimensions as may be relevant. With it, executives may move from financial accounting to 'systems accounting'. It can provide the basis for 'managerial accounting' in the sense of the managerial use not only of financial data (which is the way the term has been recently used) but of all ideas and data needed to appraise the state of a system and guide it towards the attainment of desirable future system states.[1]

---

[1]'General-systems theory' often refers to theories dealing broadly with similarities among all kinds of systems—from atoms and cells to personalities, formal organizations, and populations. In this context the term refers to a special application of general-systems theory to formal organizations—an application that deals not merely with a few aspects but generally with all aspects of formal organizations.

Before outlining a general-systems model, it is important to set aside the idea that a system is necessarily something that is fully predictable or tightly controlled. This impression is created whenever anyone tries to apply to a human organization the closed or non-human models used by physicists and engineers. A human organization is much more complicated.

Specifically, when viewed in general-systems terms, a formal organization (whether a business enterprise or a governmental agency) is

1. a man-resource system in space and time,
2. open, with various transactions between it and its environment,
3. characterized by internal and external relations of conflict as well as co-operation,
4. a system for developing and using power, with varying degrees of authority and responsibility, both within the organization and in the external environment,
5. a 'feedback' system, with information on the results of past performance activities feeding back through multiple channels to influence future performance,
6. changing, with static concepts derived from dynamic concepts rather than serving as a preliminary to them,
7. complex, that is, containing many subsystems, being contained in larger systems, and being criss-crossed by overlapping systems,
8. loose, with many components that may be imperfectly coordinated, partially autonomous, and only partially controllable,
9. only partially knowable, with many areas of uncertainty, with 'black regions' as well as 'black boxes' and with many variables that cannot be clearly defined and must be described in qualitative terms, and
10. subject to considerable uncertainty with respect to current information, future environment conditions, and the consequences of its own actions.

THE PERFORMANCE-STRUCTURE MODEL

The starting-point of modern systems analysis is the input-output concept. The flow of inputs and outputs portrays the system's performance. To apply the output concept to a formal organization, it is helpful to distinguish between two kinds of performance: producing outputs of services or goods and satisfying (or dissatisfying) various interests. To apply the input concept, a three-way breakdown is helpful: acquiring resources to be used as inputs, using inputs for investment in the system, and making efficient use of resources. In addition, we may note that organizational performance includes effort to conform with certain behaviour codes and concepts of technical and administrative rationality.

These seven kinds of performance objective may be put together in the following proposition:

> The performance of any organization or unit thereof consists of activities to (1) satisfy the varying interests of people and groups by (2) producing outputs of services or goods, (3) making efficient use of inputs relative to outputs, (4) investing in the system, (5) acquiring resources, and (6) doing all these things in a manner that conforms with various codes of behaviour and (7) varying conceptions of technical and administrative rationality.

In simplified form, the relations between these categories of performance may be visualized as follows:

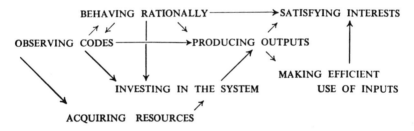

Let us now turn to system structure. The minimum elements in a machine system are certain physical components, including a 'governor' (or 'selector'), an 'effector', a 'detector', and lines of communication between them and the environment. For a formal organization these may be spelled out more specifically as subsystems in general, a central guidance subsystem, internal relations among the subsystems, and relations with the external environment. It is helpful at times to consider separately the people and the physical assets grouped together in the subsystems. It may also be helpful to give separate attention to the values held by individuals and the various subsystems.

These seven sets of structural objectives may be put together in the following proposition:

> The structure of any organization or unit thereof consists of (1) people and (2) non-human resources, (3) grouped together in differential subsystems that (4) interrelate among themselves and (5) with the external environment, (6) and are subject to various values and (7) to such central guidance as may help to provide the capacity for future performance.

In the language of matrix algebra, one can bring the two elements of system performance and system structure together into a 2 x 1 'nested' vector which may be called the 'system state vector'. Let P symbolize system performance and S system structure. Then the following sequence of vectors may symbolize changing system states over a period of time:

$$\begin{bmatrix} P \\ S \end{bmatrix}^1 \qquad \begin{bmatrix} P \\ S \end{bmatrix}^2 \qquad \dots \begin{bmatrix} P \\ S \end{bmatrix}^n$$

The vector is 'nested' because both the performance element and the structure element consist of seven subelements and are themselves 7 x 1 vectors. Each subelement, in turn, is a multidimensional matrix.

The performance vector, it should be noted, includes among its many components the basic elements in income statements and revenue-expenditure budgets. The structure vector includes all the assets (and claims against them) measured in a balance sheet. Indeed, the former may be regarded as a greatly enlarged performance budget, the latter a balance sheet that includes human and institutional assets as well as financial assets. The relations between the two are even closer than those between an income statement and a balance sheet. Almost any aspect of system performance will have some effect on system structure. Any important plans for future performance inevitably require significant changes in system structure. Changes in system structure, in turn, are invariably dependent upon some types of system performance. In everyday affairs, of course, executives often make the mistake of

—planning for major improvements in performance without giving attention to the structural prerequisites, and

—planning for major changes in structure (sometimes because of outworn or unduly abstract doctrines of formal organization) without considering their presumed connection with performance.

The skillful use of a performance-structure model may help to avoid these errors.[2]

The first elements in both structure and performance, let it be noted, are human: people and the satisfaction of people's interests. All the other elements and their many decisions—both financial and technological—are

---

[2]This performance-structure model represents a major adaptation of what has long been known as 'structural-functional' analysis. It is more dynamic than traditional structural-functional analysis, however, since it starts with action (performance) and works back to structure as the more regularized aspect of action. Also, instead of assuming a single function such as 'system maintenance', it broadens the idea of function to cover the major dimensions of performance.

ways of thinking about people and their behaviour. An organization's plans for the future are always plans made by people for people—for their future behaviour and for their future relations with resources and other people. Financial and technological planners may easily lose sight of these human elements. Another virtue of general-systems analysis, therefore, is that it helps to bring together the 'soft' information of human relations people with the 'hard' data of accountants and engineers.

PERFORMANCE OBJECTIVES

Any of the seven elements of system performance, as baldly stated above, may be used in a statement of 'where we want to go' or as a criterion of 'doing an effective job'. But none of them is meaningful unless broken down into its subelements. When this is done, indeed, the basic subelements may be rearranged in many ways. There is no magic in any one ordering.

Within the present space limits I shall merely touch upon some of the major dimensions of each element and subelement. Additional details are available in *The Managing of Organizations* (Gross, 1964, Pt. V, Chs. 20–29).

Some random illustrations for both an organization (an aircraft company) and a unit thereof (its personnel office) are provided in *Table 1*. *Tables 2* and *3* provide more detailed illustrations in two areas of special complexity: output objectives and input-output objectives. In these tables 'goal' refers to a specific type of subelement and 'norm' to a more specific formulation of a goal. To save space, reference to the tables will not be made in the text.

1. Satisfying Interests

Although the satisfaction of human interests is the highest purpose of any organization, interest-satisfaction objectives (often referred to as *benefits, welfare, utility, value,* or *payoff*) are the most difficult to formulate.

First of all, such objectives always involve a multiplicity of parties at interest—or 'interesteds'. These include the members of the organization, the organization's 'clientele network', and other external groups and individuals. They vary considerably in visibility and in the extent to which their interests are affected by an organization's performance.

Second, their interests are usually multiple, often hard to identify, always divergent, and sometimes sharply conflicting. In psychological terms these interests may be described in terms of the human needs for security, belonging, status, prestige, power, and self-development. Many

Table 1. Performance Objectives: Some General Illustrations

Performance Objectives	Aircraft Company		Personnel Unit	
	Goals	Norms	Goals	Norms
1. Satisfying Interests				
(a) Members	Higher morale	Reducing labor turnover to 6%	Professional prestige	Leadership in professional organizations
(b) Clientele network	Meeting airlines' needs	5% rise in total sales	Meeting needs of line	Fewer complaints
(c) Others	Investors	Maintaining 3% yield on common stock	Serving all employees	Reducing labor turnover to 10%
2. Producing Output				
(a) Output mix	Adding short-range jets	End-product production schedule	New management training program	End-product services
(b) Quantity	Increased market penetration	15% of industry sales	Greater coverage	150 'trainees' per year
(c) Quality	Safer planes	Wing improvements	Better designed courses	Better consultants
(d) Output flow	Work-flow	Detailed schedules	Work-flow	Detailed schedules
3. Making Efficient Use of Inputs				
(a) Profitability	Higher profits on net worth (or total assets)	20% on net worth	—	—
(b) Costs per unit	Lower engine costs	8% reduction	Total costs per trainee	$200 per week
(c) Partial input ratios	More output per man-hour	10% increase	Teacher costs	$150 per training-hour
(d) Portion of potential used	Reducing idle equipment-time	5% reduction	Full participation in program	No vacancies

4. Investing in the Organization			
(a) Hard goods	Re-equipment program	Detailed specifications	New files	No vacancies
(b) People	Management training program	50 trainees per year	'Retooling' of old-timers	Participation in 'refresher' courses
(c) Internal units	Reorganization of personnel unit	Higher status for training section	Maintenance of existing organization	Maintaining present status for training section
(d) External relations	More support in Congress	Support by specific senators	More support from 'line' executives	Support by specific executives
5. Acquiring Resources			
(a) Money	More equity	Selling securities	Larger budget	5% increase
(b) People	Better managers	Recruitment program	More professional staff	Recruitment program
(c) Goods	New machines	Procurement program	New files	Procurement program
6. Observing Codes			
(a) External codes	Obeying anti-trust laws	Competition within limits	Living within budgets	Controls on commitments
(b) Internal codes	Obeying company regs.	Control of deviations	Loyalty to unit	Social exclusiveness
7. Behaving Rationally			
(a) Technical rationality	Aeronautical research	Specific studies	Personnel research	Specific studies
(b) Administrative rationality	Formal reorganization	More decentralization	More 'democracy'	Monthly staff meetings

Table 2. Output Performance Objectives: Some Detailed Illustrations

Output Production Objectives	Aircraft Company		Personnel Unit	
	Goals	Norms	Goals	Norms
A. Output Mix	Continued output of long-range jets New short-range jet Parts production Research for government Advisory services for users	Detailed production schedule	Maintaining personnel records Recruitment services Classification system Job analysis and evaluation Training program	Operating program
B. Output Quality				
1. Client satisfactions				
(a) Presumed results	Planes: Faster, safer flights	Specific speed and safety standards	Training program: Better managers	Subsequent performance of trainees
(b) Choices made	Popularity among passengers	Prosperity of airline customers	Popularity of program	Backlog of applicants
(c) Payments given	Rising volume of airline sales	15% of industry sales	Budgets allocated	Specific budget figures
(d) Opinions expressed	Low complaint level	Decline in pilots' complaints	Trainees' opinions	Specific statements
2. Product characteristics	Conformance with specifications	Detailed specifications	Improved curriculum	Emphasis on decision-skills
3. Production processes	Careful testing	Specific tests	Improved teaching methods	Use of field studies
4. Input quality	Outstanding productive personnel	Acquiring best designers	Outstanding teachers	Acquiring teachers of repute

C. Output Quantity

1. Monetary value			
(a) Total sales value	Planes: 15% of industry sales	X million dollars	—
(b) Value added	Lower proportion of value added with more sub-contracting	$\dfrac{X}{3}$	—
(c) Value added adjusted for price changes	20% beyond 1960	$\dfrac{X \cdot 9}{3}$ (price deflator)	—
(d) Imputed values of nonmarketed output	Advisory services: Input value	Specific cost figures	Specific cost figures
2. Physical volume			
(a) Tangible units	Planes: Number to be produced	Detailed production schedule	—
(b) Surrogates for in-tangible services	Advisory services:		Input value
(i) clients	More clients	⎫	Training program:
(ii) duration	Longer periods	⎬ Specific figures	⎫ More trainees
(iii) intermediate or subsequent products	Memoranda produced	⎭	⎬ Longer courses
			⎭ Field studies undertaken
			Specific figures
(iv) input value	Total costs	Total costs	—

Table 3. Input-Output Performance Objectives: Some Detailed Illustrations

Efficiency (Input-Output) Objectives	Aircraft Company Goals	Aircraft Company Norms	Personnel Unit Goals	Personnel Unit Norms
A. Profitability				
1. Unit profits	Short-range jet; higher profits with rising volume	Specific figures	—	—
2. Total profits				
Before taxes	Higher profits	10% increase		
After taxes	Higher profits	12% increase	—	—
Total profits	Lower (with replacement of debt by equity)	10% decrease		
3. Net worth	Higher	10% increase	—	—
4. Total assets		10% increase	—	—
5. Sales	Lower (with higher volume of sales)	10% decrease	—	—
B. Costs per Unit	New short-range jets: Declining total costs with rising volume	10% decline per unit over first year	Training program: Rising costs with longer duration and higher quality	20% more per trainee
C. Partial Input-Output Relations				
1. Labor-output ratios				
(a) Labor time	For a specific output unit: More output per direct man-hour	10% increase	More teacher-time per trainee	10% more per trainee

(b) Labor cost	No increase in direct costs Small increase in direct plus indirect labor costs	Same 5% increase	Higher teacher fees Higher overhead costs	20% more per trainee 5% increase
(c) Output per $1 of labor cost	Lower total value Lower added value	-6% -29%	— —	— —
2. Capital-output ratio	For specific machines; fuller use of rated capacity	Specific figures	Low-cost residential facilities	Specific figures
D. Portion of Output Potential Used				
1. Waste	Less scrap material Better utilization of scrap Fuller use of capacity	Specific figures Reaching 80% in 2 shifts	Less waste Fuller use of computers (on personnel records)	Elimination of unnecessary paperwork Reaching 35% of capacity
2. Gap between actual potential	Higher fulfilment of profit potential	8% on total assets	Higher fulfilment of potential	Specific data on quality quantity of end-products

Table 4. Structural Objectives: Some General Illustrations

Structural Objectives	Aircraft Company		Personnel Unit	
	Goals	Norms	Goals	Norms
1. People				
(a) Types	Fewer 'blue-collars'	Specific manning tables	More professionals	Specific manning tables
(b) Quantity	No overall increase	Specific manning tables	Larger staff	4 new positions
(c) Quality	Better-educated staff	90% college graduates above supervisory level	Better educational back-ground	All college graduates with a few PhDs
2. Non-human resources				
(a) Physical assets	More modern plant	Specific re-equipment program	More adequate space	5 more rooms
(b) Monetary assets	More liquid position	2 : 1 current liability ratio	Larger reserves	More transferable budget items
(c) Claims against assets	Higher ratio of equity to long-term debt	$10 million equity increase	—	—
3. Subsystems				
(a) Units	Improved divisional structure	Stronger jet-plane divisions	Improved internal structure	Stronger training group
(b) Committees	Improved committee structure	Inter-divisional task force on new jets	Better representation on committees	Participation in jet-plane task force
4. Subsystem relations				
(a) Cooperation-conflict	Settlement of inter-divisional disputes	Compromise on jet-plane design	Settlement of inter-unit disputes	Compromise on location of training division
(b) Hierarchy	Stronger central control	Fewer levels	Stronger unit position	Direct line to top manager
(c) Polyarchy	Dispersed responsibility	New clearance procedures	Dispersed responsibility	New clearance procedures
(d) Communication	Better communication among divisions	Weekly paper	Better communication with line executives	Liaison units in line divisions

5. External relations				
(a) Clients and suppliers	Better distribution channels for parts	Relations with specific distributors	More supports from line executives	Support by specific executives
(b) Controllers and controllees	More support in Congress	Support by specific Senators	More support by budget unit	Support for 4 new positions
(c) Associates and adversaries	Limits on competition	'Understandings' on division of markets	Rivalry with budget unit	Less budget opposition to training program funds
6. Values				
(a) Internal-external orientation	Public service	Safer planes	Professionalism in personnel management	Advancement of unit's interests
(b) Conformity and individualism	Initiative	Proposing of company policy by divisions	Loyalty to unit	Subordination of external interests
(c) Activism-passivity	Progress	Faster planes	Progress	All-round improvement
7. System management				
(a) Higher level	More 'professional' approach	Specific planning and control methods	More 'human' approach	More emphasis on personnel management
(b) Lower level	More effective supervision	Participatory activation methods	More effective supervision	Better check of supervisors

of these needs are expressed in terms of services and goods designed to meet them and the monetary income which, in a market economy, is necessary to provide such services and goods. They may also be expressed in terms of the needs for both employment and leisure. The terms 'public interest' or 'national interest' are ways of referring to the great multiplicity of interests that many people and groups throughout a society have in common. There are always conflicting views concerning the nature of 'public interests'.

Third, it is immensely difficult to specify the extent of satisfactions desired or attained. Satisfactions themselves are locked in the hearts and minds of the people whose interests are presumed to be satisfied. They are inextricably associated with dissatisfactions and frustration. The most we can do is use certain indirect indicators expressed in terms of the observable behaviour of the behaviour of 'interesteds'. Two of the most immediate forms of behaviour are the choices they make (in participating in the organization or using its product) and money they are willing to pay (in the form of consumer purchases, taxes, or dues). Other indicators are their expressed opinions (complaints or praise) and their subsequent behaviour as a presumed result of the satisfactions obtained. Such indicators with respect to clientele satisfactions provide the most important measures of output quality.

2. Producing Output

Output production objectives are much easier to formulate. They may best be expressed in terms of an 'output mix' listing the types of services or goods supplied to the organization's (or unit's) clientele. For each type quality and quantity objectives may then be set.

Yet there are at least five major problems in this area. First of all, output quality has many dimensions. As already indicated, clientele satisfaction, the most important dimension of output quality, is exceedingly difficult to measure. Less direct indicators—such as product specifications, production processes, and the quality of input factors—may also be needed. The objective of higher quality often conflicts with the objective of higher quantity.

Second, although monetary aggregates are the only way of measuring total output, they must be used with considerable care. Important distinctions may be needed between the total value of output and value added, between marginal value and total or average value, between different ways of allocating value to time periods. For comparisons over time, adjustments for price changes may be needed; for international comparisons, adjustments in the value of international currencies.

Third, in the case of services and goods that are not sold (and this includes most of the intermediate output within business organizations) the only direct measure of output quantity is physical units. In most instances this means that there is no common denominator for the total quantity of different kinds of unit. All that can be done to aggregate quantity objectives is to use input costs or some administratively determined 'price' (as an internal pricing systems) as an indirect quantity indicator.

Fourth, in the case of intangible services there are no physical units that can readily be identified. Here one can set objectives only in terms of such indirect indicators as the number of clients, the duration of services, certain intermediate products that are more tangible, and the volume or value of input factors.

Fifth, considerable confusion may develop between intermediate products and the end-products supplied to an organization's clientele. This readily happens with intangible end-product services that are provided on a non-sale basis to an intangible, unorganized, or reluctant clientele. More tangible intermediate products—particularly when supplied by hard-driving, ambitious units—may then receive disproportionate attention. One remedy is to formulate objectives in terms of work-flow—that is, a series of intermediate outputs leading to the production of the organization's end-products.

3. Making Efficient Use of Inputs

When resources available for use as inputs are perceived as scarce, an organization or unit usually becomes interested in making efficient use of inputs relative to outputs. Since there are many ways of calculating input and output and of relating the two, there are many varieties of input-output performance.

Profitability is the most useful input-output relation, since it provides a common measure for value for both input and output. Profitability measures may be used in many ways, however, depending upon whether one (1) relates profits to net worth, total assets, or sales (2) focuses on unit profits or total profits, or (3) thinks in short- or long-range terms. Depending upon a variety of techniques for handling difficult accounting problems, they are subject to considerable statistical manipulation. They may also reflect an organization's monopoly power and its ability to obtain subsidies, as well as its efficiency. Nevertheless, in many circumstances—particularly over a long time period—profitability is the best single measure of efficiency, output quantity and quality, and interest satisfaction.

The most generally applicable efficiency objective is attaining the lowest possible total costs for a given unit of output. This cost-accounting measure is an essential instrument in attaining—even in formulating—profitability objectives. It is relevant to non-marketed products as well. In developing cost-accounting goals, however, it is essential not to neglect the quality dimensions of output. In the case of intangible services, as already indicated, the identification of the unit is extremely difficult. Where capital and material inputs are involved, it is necessary to make difficult—and sometimes arbitrary—decisions with respect to depreciation, the distinction between current and capital expenditures, and the value of withdrawals from inventories.

Partial input-output ratios are those relating some measure of input—usually either labour or capital—to some measure of total output. Such a ratio is particularly meaningful when the volume of other input factors may be presumed to remain unchanged. It will be very misleading, however, whenever there is any significant change in any other input factor—as when increased output per employee is counterbalanced, and in fact caused, by increased capital per unit of output.

Another efficiency measure is the proportion of potential actually used. This may be expressed in terms of a reduction in waste, a higher utilization of capacity (potential output), or profits in relation to potential profitability.

4. Investing in the System

In addition to producing current output, an organization must invest in its capacity for future production. Investment objectives involve the expansion, replacement, conservation, or development of assets. They are essential not only for survival, but to prevent decline or promote growth.

The most obvious investment objectives relate to hard goods and monetary reserves. The hard goods may include land, buildings, equipment and machinery, and stocks of materials. The monetary reserves may include cash, deposits, securities, receivables, and any other funds that can be drawn upon.

Less obvious, although equally important, is investment in people, subsystems, subsystem relations, external relations, and the development of values. Investment in the guidance subsystem itself—that is, in the management structure—is particularly important.

In other words, investment performance may deal directly with any element of system structure. Accordingly, the specifics of investment objectives may be presented in the subsequent discussion of system structure.

In general, however, it should be pointed out that investment objectives often mean a diversion of resources from use in current output. Thus there are often important conflicts not only among different forms of investment but between investment and output production.

5. Acquiring Resources

Neither output production nor investment is possible without resources that can be used as inputs. These must be obtained from the external environment or from within the organization. Under conditions of scarcity and competition this requires considerable effort. Thus resource-acquisition objectives usually receive high priority. Indeed, long-range planning is often oriented much more to acquiring resources than to utilizing them.

Organizations that sell their output may acquire external resources from the consumer market (through sales revenue), the capital market (through investment), and banks (through loans). Their sales, investment, and borrowing objectives are closely related to the extent of clientele satisfactions. Organizations and units that do not sell their output must depend mainly upon budgetary allocations.

In both cases monetary terms provide the most general expression of resource-mobilization objectives. But the monetary objectives are meaningful only when they reflect the specific resources to be acquired with money—people, information, facilities, goods, or organizations. In many circumstances it is also necessary to include (1) specifications for the resources desired, (2) specific terms and conditions, (3) selection methods, (4) the maintenance of supply lines, and (5) inspection of resources received.

The logical justification of an organization's 'requirements' for additional resources is best provided by a set of objectives that moves back from (1) interest satisfactions and (2) output mix to (3) efficiency and (4) investment. In the budget-allocation process 'acquisition logic' also requires efforts to appeal to the interests of those with most influence in the allocation decisions.

6. Observing Codes

Every organization aims at doing things in the 'right' way. To some extent the 'right' way is set forth in external codes—laws, regulations, moral and ethical prohibitions and prescriptions, and professional principles. It is also determined by the codes of the organization—its written and unwritten rules and rituals.

Some may prefer to think of code observance as a restraint upon efforts to attain other objectives. None the less, a considerable amount of purposeful activity in organizations is involved in containing inevitable tendencies towards code deviation.

The greatest attention is usually given to internal codes. In the case of external codes that are not 'internalized', the organization will often tolerate deviation. Indeed, the deception of external inspectors may itself become part of the internal code. Similarly, the deception of the organization's code-enforcement efforts may become part of the internal code of various units. These tendencies towards deviation are facilitated by the difficulty of understanding—or even keeping up with—complex regulations. They are promoted by recurring code conflicts.

These difficulties may be handled only in part by formal enforcement measures. Successful code observance also requires widespread internalization of codes and the continuing adjustment of conflicting and confusing codes.

7. Behaving Rationally

An organization or unit also aims at doing things 'rationally'. This means the selection of the most satisfactory means of attaining a given set of objectives—from interest satisfaction and output production down to rational behaviour itself. Thus rationality is an all-pervasive instrumental objective.

Perfect rationality is an impossible objective. The instruments of rational calculation—information, knowledge, and skill—are always imperfect. The dimensions of rational behaviour—desirability, feasibility, and consistency—are themselves frequently conflicting. The more desirable objective will frequently be less feasible, the more feasible objective less consistent with other goals, the more consistent objective less desirable.

Technical rationality involves the use of the best methods devised by science and technology. With rapid scientific and technological progress, it is constantly changing. On the one hand, the rational methods of a few years ago may be irrational today. On the other hand, new techniques are often adapted on the basis of 'technological faddism' rather than truly rational choice. In either case, there are usually serious disputes among technicians, disputes that cannot be entirely settled within the confines of technical rationality.

Administrative rationality is a much broader type of rationality. It involves the use of the best methods of guiding or managing organizations. This involves the interrelated processes of planning, activating, and evaluating with respect to all significant dimensions of both performance and structure. It provides the framework for resolving technical disputes. Yet administrative rationality, although highly developed on an intuitive basis, still awaits systematic scientific formulation. Many so-called 'principles' of administration neglect the major dimensions of performance, deal formalistically with structure, and ignore the relation between the two.

Management theory has not yet gone far enough in encouraging managers to think and communicate explicitly in connexion with such delicate subjects as the development and use of power and the management of internal and external conflict.

STRUCTURE OBJECTIVES

In thinking of system structure we should beware of images derived from the 'non-human' structure of a building. The structure of an organization is based upon the expectations and behavior of people and human groups. It has informal as well as formal aspects. It can never be understood (not even in its formal aspects) from an inspection of written decisions alone. It is never free from internal conflicts and inconsistencies. Unlike the frame of a building, it is always changing in many ways. Indeed, structure is merely the more stabilized aspect of activity. It consists of interrelations that provide the capacity for future performance and that can be understood only in terms of performance objectives. Some random illustrations of objectives for structural change are provided in *Table 4*.

1. People

The people in an organization are the first element in an organization's structure. Thus structural objectives may be formulated in terms of the types of personnel, their quality, and their quantity.

Personnel may be classified in terms of specific positions with such-and-such titles, salaries, and perquisites; abilities, knowledge, and interests; experience; educational background; health; and various personality characteristics. Other characteristics relate to age, sex, race, religion, geographical origins. Some combination of these dimensions is usually employed in objectives for recruitment, replacement, and promotion.

The formulation of quality objectives involves consideration of the place of various people within a specific subsystem. Without reference to any subsystem, however, it also involves attention to people's capacity for learning and self-development. It involves objectives for promoting the utilization of such capacity.

The number of people in an organization is one of the simplest measures of its size. Larger numbers are often sought as a prelude to obtaining other assets, as a substitute for them, or as compensation for the lack of quality. Even with high-quality personnel and an adequate complement of non-human resources, larger numbers are often needed to supply essential reserves or the basis of major output expansion.

2. Non-human Resources

With advancing science and technology, non-human resources become increasingly essential as instruments of human activity.

Certain natural resources—if only a piece of land—are an essential foundation of human activity. Physical facilities provide the necessary housing for human activity. Equipment and machinery, particularly when driven by electrical energy, make it possible for people to move or process things with little expenditure of human energy. Data-processing machinery replaces human labour in the processing of information. Thus investment objectives must deal with the structure of these physical assets.

As indicated in the discussion of investment performance, they may also include objectives with respect to monetary assets and—where balance-sheet accounting is used—to the structure of claims against them (liabilities).

3. Subsystems

Within any organization people and non-human resources are grouped together in various subsystems. Each subsystem, in turn, is often subdivided still further. The smallest subdivision is the individual person.

Each subsystem is identifiable mainly by its role or function. The major element in role definition is the output expected from the subsystem. In larger organizations, particularly those based upon advancing technology, role differentiation tends to become increasingly specific and detailed. It also tends to undergo change—but at uneven and varying rates in response to recurring new environmental conditions, new technology, and adjustments in the quantity and quality of the organization's output mix. This means an internal restructuring of the subsystems. With growth of the organization as a whole, the subsystems change in a disproportional manner. Some expand, some decline, and some must be liquidated.

Important distinctions must be made between individuals and roles. People may come and go, while a role remains. Moreover, one person may play a number of roles—that is, 'wear many hats'. Some roles are substantially developed by the people who play them. Most people are substantially affected by the roles they play.

There are many kinds of subsystem. Some are hierarchically organized units; others are committees. Some are organized to perform functions peculiar to a specific organization; others provide certain kinds of services (personnel, budgeting, accounting, procurement, methods analysis, public relations) that are widely used by many organizations. Some are called 'line', others 'staff'. Some are informal only. The most important subsystem is the management or guidance subsystem (discussed separately under 7 below).

4. Internal Relations

By itself subsystem differentiation is divisive. The system as a whole exists only to the extent that the parts are brought together in a network of internal relations.

The first element in internal relations is cooperation among and within the subsystems. This cooperation must be based upon certain commonly accepted objectives for future performance. Otherwise work-flows will not mesh. A large part of this cooperation may consist of routinized, habitual expectations and activity. At the same time cooperation is always associated with conflict relations within and among subsystems. If carried too far, conflict and tension may impair—even destroy—the internal structure. Within limits they may help to invigorate it.

Hierarchic relations are an indispensable element in the cooperation-conflict nexus. These consist of superior-subordinate relations, usually confined to certain spheres of behaviour. The lines of hierarchic authority provide formal channels of internal communication and ladders for career advancement. The upper positions in a hierarchy provide valuable points for conflict settlement and important symbols of organizational unity. At the same time, the growing role differentiation in modern organizations leads inevitably towards the subdivision of hierarchic authority and the growth of 'multiple hierarchy' (see Gross, 1964, pp. 377–9).

Hierarchy is always accompanied by polyarchy—sometimes referred to as 'lateral relations'. One form of polyarchy is 'joint authority'. Thus committee members (often representing different units) may operate together as equals rather than as superiors and subordinates. Another is 'dispersed authority'. In budget procedures various units negotiate and bargain with each other—at least up to the point where hierarchic authority may be brought into play.

The communication network is an all-pervasive part of internal relations. A critical role in this network is always played by the various lines of hierarchic authority. But many other multi-directional channels and media—some of them informal—are also needed.

5. External Relations

The immediate environment of any organization includes not only individuals but also various groups that may be classified as enterprises, government agencies, and various types of association. The relations between an organization and this immediate environment may be expressed in terms of the roles played by such individuals and groups:

(a) Clients and suppliers
The clients are those who receive, or are supposed to benefit from, an organization's output. The suppliers are those who supply the goods, services, information, or money acquired by the organization.

(b) Controllers and controllees
The controllers are the external regulators or 'superiors'. The controllees are the organization's regulatees or 'subordinates'.

(c) Associates and adversaries
The associates are partners or allies engaged in joint or cooperative undertakings. The adversaries include rivals for the same resources, competitors in producing similar outputs, and outright enemies interested in limiting or destroying the organization's performance or structure.

The same external organization often plays many—at times even all—of these roles. In so doing it will use many forms of external persuasion, pressure, or penetration.

Resistance to external influence usually involves an organization in preventive or counter measures of persuasion, pressure, or penetration. A more positive approach to external relations involves efforts to isolate, neutralize, or win over opponents and build up a farflung structure of external support through coalitions, alliances, and 'deals'. Such efforts may be facilitated by persuasive efforts aimed at unorganized publics.

6. Values

The individuals and subsystems in any organization are always guided by some pattern of values—that is, general attitudes towards what is desirable or undesirable and general ways of looking at the world. Some of the most important elements in this value structure may be defined in terms of the continua between

(a) Internal and external orientation
Internal orientation emphasizes the interests of members—in terms of their income, status, power, or self-development. External orientation emphasizes the interests of non-members; these may range from investors (owners) to clients to the society as a whole. Some organizations aim at integrating the two sets of values.

(b) Conformity and individualism

In many organizations conformity is a high value—sometimes to the point of the complete subordination of individual initiative. Nevertheless, highly individualistic values may be hidden behind a façade of superficial conformism.

(c) Passivity and activism

Among many members or organizations passivity is a highly cherished value. It leads to 'playing it safe', 'taking it easy', 'following the book', and waiting for orders. Activist values, in contrast, lead to risk-taking, initiative, and innovation. Although apparently conflicting, the two are often intertwined.

Other values relate to freedom and control, authoritarianism and democracy, material and non-material interests, equity and equality, impersonality and particularism, and ascription and achievement.

7. Guidance Subsystem

Some amount of coordinated action is always provided by the autonomous action—both routinized and spontaneous—of an organization's subsystems. But sufficient capacity for effective performance is not possible without the coordinating and promotional functions of a special subsystem with the responsibility for system guidance, or management. This guidance subsystem is composed of a network extending from a general directorate and top executives down through the middle and lower levels of managerial or supervisory personnel. At any level the members of this subsystem play various roles in decision-making and communication with respect to the making of plans, the activating of people and groups, and the evaluating of plans made and action taken. The interrelation among these roles helps to determine the structure of the guidance subsystem.

An important aspect of management structure is the balance between centralization and decentralization. Both centralization and decentralization may be thought of in terms of the distribution of responsibility and authority by (a) vertical levels, (b) horizontal levels, and (c) geographical location. The extent of centralization or decentralization in any of these dimensions can best be specified with reference to specific roles or functions. The prerequisite for effective decentralization of some functions is the centralization of other functions. With increasing size and complexity, it usually becomes necessary to delegate greater responsibility and authority to lower levels and to field offices. This, in turn, requires the strengthening of certain planning, activating, and evaluating functions *of* the 'centre', as well as various horizontal shifts in the centralization-decentralization balance *in* the centre.

Another vital aspect of management structure is its power base. This includes the resources at its disposal. It includes the support it obtains from the membership and major points of internal influence. It includes the support obtained externally—from associates, from clients and suppliers, and from controllers and controllees. Top business executives need support from their boards of directors and banks; government executives from President or Governor, legislators, and external interest groups.

Other important dimensions of management structure relate to managerial personnel and tenure. Admission to the upper ranks of management may be dependent upon a combination of such factors as sponsorship, ability, education, personality characteristics, and social origins. Some top managers seek a self-perpetuating oligarchy, with little or no provision made for inevitable replacement. Others set as major objectives the development of career and recruitment systems that make for high mobility within managerial ranks.

THE STRATEGY OF PLANNING

Planning is the process of developing commitments to some pattern of objectives.

The preceding section set forth the major categories of objectives.

Let us now turn to some of the strategic considerations involved in deriving a pattern from these categories.

1. The Selectivity Paradox

As specialists develop comprehensive ways of looking at systems, they often tend to overemphasize the role of comprehensive objectives in planning. Thus economists often give the false impression that national aggregates of income, product, investment, and consumption are the major goals in national policy-making. In the process of 'selling their wares', budgeteers and accountants often give the impression that comprehensive projections of budgets, income statements, or balance sheets can define an organization's major goals. If this approach should be automatically transferred to general-systems accounting, we should then find ourselves recommending that an organization's planners should formulate comprehensive objectives for all the elements of system performance and system structure.

Yet this would be a misleading position. The essence of planning is the *selection of strategic objectives in the form of specific sequences of action to be taken by the organization.* These critical variables must be selected in terms of:

(a) The major interest satisfactions that must be 'promised' to obtain external and internal support.

(b) Present, imminent, or foreseeable crises or emergencies. These may require 'contingency plans'.

(c) Their decisive impact upon preceding, coordinate, or subsequent events.

(d) The long-range implications of action in the present or the immediate future. These are the critical considerations with respect to the 'sunk costs' of investment programmes and the immediate steps in extended production processes (such as the building of houses, ships, or aircraft).

With these strategic elements selected, many elements of performance and structure may be detailed in subsystem plans or handled on the basis of current improvisation. A passion for comprehensive detail by either the organization or its subsystems may undermine selectivity. It may easily result in a loss of perspective, in document-orientation instead of action-orientation, and in an information supply that overloads communication channels and processing capacity. It may thus lead to serious waste of resources.

But—and here is the paradox of selectivity—strategic objectives can be selected rationally *only if the planners are aware of the broad spectrum of possible objectives.* Otherwise, objectives may be set in a routinized, arbitrary, or superficial fashion. The very concept of selection implies the scanning of a broad range of possibilities.

The solution to this paradox may be found in the use of general-systems accounting to provide a *comprehensive background for the selection of strategic objectives.*

2. The Clarity-Vagueness Balance

There is no need to labour the need for clarity in the formulation of an organization's objectives. Precise formulations are necessary for delicate operations. They provide the indispensable framework for coordinating complex activity. They often have great symbolic significance.

Yet in the wide enthusiasm for 'crystal-clear goals', one may easily lose sight of the need for a fruitful balance between clarity and vagueness. The following quotation is an effort to contribute to this balance through a 'crystal-clear' statement on the virtues of vagueness:

If all the points on a set of interrelated purpose chains were to be set forth with precise clarity, the result would be to destroy the subordination of one element to another which is essential to an operating purpose pattern. The proper focusing of attention on some goals for any particular moment or period in time means that other goals must be left vague. This is even more true for different periods of time. We must be very clear about many things we aim to do today and tomorrow. It might be dangerously misleading to seek similar clarity for our long-range goals.

Apart from its role in helping provide focus, vagueness in goal formation has many positive virtues. It leaves room for others to fill in the details and even modify the general pattern; over-precise goals stifle initiative. Vagueness may make it easier to adapt to changing conditions; ultra-precision can destroy flexibility. Vagueness may make it possible to work towards many goals that can only be attained by indirection. Some of the deepest personal satisfactions from work and cooperation come as by-products of other things. If pursued too directly, they may slip through one's fingers; the happiest people in the world are never those who set out to do the things that will make them happy. There is something inhuman and terrifying about ultrapurposeful action proceeding according to blueprint and schedule. Only vagueness can restore the precious element of humanity.

Above all, vagueness is an essential part of all agreements resulting from compromise. When a dispute is resolved, some degree of ambiguity enters into the terms of settlement. Hence the wide-open language often used in the final language of statutory law. Similar ambiguities are found in most constitutions, charters, declarations of purpose, policy manifestos, and collective bargaining agreements. Certain anticipated situations are always referred to in terms that mean different things to different people, and are valuable because of, not despite, this characteristic. (Gross, 1964, p. 497.)

3. Whose Objectives?

Whose objectives are an organization's objectives?

The crystal-clear answers to this question point to (1) the people who wrote the charter (law or articles of incorporation) under which the organization operates, (2) the holders of formal authority over the organization (legislators or stockholders), (3) the members of the organization as a whole, (4) the organization's specialized planning people, or (5) the organization's top managers.

Yet each of these answers is incomplete. The charter-writers and the holders of formal authority can deal with only a small portion of an organization's objectives. The members, the subsystems, and the specialized planners have or propose many objectives that the organization never accepts. The managers' objectives may be accepted only in part by the rest of the organization. All of these groups have many conflicting objectives.

A better, although vaguer, answer is one that defines an organization's objectives as those widely accepted by its members. These objectives may (to some extent, they *must*) reflect the objectives of charter-writers, the holders of formal authority, and other external groups. They must represent a common area of acceptance on the part of the organization's subsystems and members, albeit within a matrix of divergent and conflicting purposes. The technical planners play a major role in helping to formulate planning decisions. The top managers make (or legitimate) the decisions and play a major role in winning their acceptance throughout the organization. Whether recognized in formal planning procedures or not, the entire management structure is involved *de facto* in the daily operation of formulating and winning commitment to objectives for future performance and structure.

4. Conflict Resolving and Creating

As already indicated, the process of organizational planning involves dealing with many conflicting objectives and with divergent or conflicting parties at interest both inside and outside an organization.

Hence planning—rather than involving nothing but the sober application of technical rationality—is an exercise in conflict management. In this exercise systematic technical calculations are exceedingly valuable as a means both of narrowing areas of conflict and of revealing possibilities for conflict resolution. Yet technical calculations are never enough. Over-reliance upon them can lead to administrative irrationality.

Rational planning, in contrast, requires realistic attention to the power for and against alternative plans. It requires the resolution of conflicts through the use of power in various combinations of persuasion and pressure. It also requires the building of a power base through various methods of conflict resolution.

The most widespread mode of conflict resolution is compromise, through which some interests are sacrificed. A more creative—but more difficult—method is integration. This involves a creative readjustment of interests so that all parties may gain and none lose. In some cases, total victory may be obtained for one point of view, with consequent defeat for its opposition. To prevent defeat on some objectives, it is often necessary to tolerate deadlock or avoid an issue entirely. Any real-life planning process may be characterized as a *stream of successive compromises punctuated by frequent occasions of deadlock or avoidance and occasional victories, defeats, and integrations.* All these outcomes lead to new conflicts to be handled by the planners and managers.

Successful planning is often possible only when the key members of an organization see themselves threatened by an imminent crisis. In non-crisis conditions the subsystems tend to move in their own directions. They will most readily accept common objectives when the alternative is perceived as an onslaught of acute dissatisfactions, that is, a crisis. With crisis as the alternative, conflicts may be more quickly and effectively resolved. This is particularly relevant to subsystem resistance against plans for significant structural change.

In developing an organization's purposes, therefore, managers are frequently involved in crisis management. They try to anticipate crises around the corner. They try to respond promptly to crises that emerge. They may even try to create crises by setting high aspirations and accentuating fears of failure. These are delicate activities. For managers without a broad perspective on an organization's performance, structure, and environmental relations, they are dangerous undertakings—with much to be lost on one front as the price of victory on another. Even with such a broad perspective, they involve considerations that may not always be publicly discussed with complete frankness.

Hence a better-developed language of organizational purposefulness will not provide an outsider with a satisfactory answer when he asks a manager, 'Just what are your organization's purposes?' The most it can do is help the managers themselves in the difficult and unending process of asking the question and finding workable answers.

References

Drucker, Peter F. (1954). *The practice of management.* New York: Harper.

Drucker, Peter F. (1964). *Managing for results.* New York: Harper & Row.

Gross, Bertram M. (1964). *The managing of organizations* (2 vols). New York: Free Press.

LeBreton, Preston P. & Henning, Dale A. (1961). *Planning theory.* Englewood Cliffs, N.J.: Prentice-Hall.

CHAPTER 5

DECISION-MAKING

A *decision* is the conclusion of a process designed to weigh the relative utilities of a set of available alternatives so that the most preferred course of action can be selected for implementation. *Decision-making* involves all the thinking and activities that are required to identify the most preferred choice. In particular, the making of a decision requires a set of goals and objectives; a system of priorities; an enumeration of alternative courses of feasible and viable actions; the projection of consequences associated with different alternatives; and a system of choice criteria by which the most preferred course is identified. Decision-making is a *pervasive, deliberative, continuous, constant,* and *sequential* activity.

Its *pervasive* nature is obvious from the fact that all of us are engaged in the making and implementation of decisions in various roles that we accept in life. The *deliberative* nature of decision-making is important because it implies an approach based on thought and reflection—as opposed to actions arising from habit and reflex. Decision-making is also a *continuous* as well as a *constant* process because all human actions are related, in

223

one form or the other, to the making and implementation of decisions. Although it is possible to analyze the making of a specific decision as an isolated phenomenon, decisions are essentially *sequential* in nature. The sequential nature of decisions is obvious from the fact that in the interdependent world of today each decision has consequences and implications far beyond its original boundaries drawn under simplifying assumptions.

Decision theory, the body of knowledge that deals with the analysis and making of decisions, is an important area of study. Decision theory deals with the analysis and making of decisions under specified conditions, such as risk and uncertainty. Such diverse disciplines as philosophy, economics, psychology, sociology, statistics, political science, and operations research have made significant contributions to the area of decision theory. We can identify several different approaches to the study of decision-making. One relates to the preliminary questions of *how* to formulate goals and objectives, enumerate environmental constraints, identify alternative strategies, and project relevant payoffs. The second concentrates on the question of how to choose the optimal strategy when we are given a set of objectives, strategies, and payoffs. Both of these approaches are important to administrators, and, in practice, the two are intertwined.

The process of choosing the optimal strategy has been made more efficient by the development of quantitative decision models. Some of these models are described in Selection 15. In each and every decision situation, regardless of its content or orientation, a sequence of eight steps must be executed—explicitly or implicitly. These steps constitute the basic structure of a decision model which is enclosed within the dotted lines as shown in Figure 5.1.

Formulation of objectives and goals, the *first* step in our model, is usually preceded by a series of activities which are often referred to as *perception* and *intelligence*. The essential purpose of these activities is to define the problem. The purpose of the *second* step is to "take stock" of the prevailing circumstances. In particular, the manager lists his resources; the constraints that delimit his freedom of action; future anticipated economic, political, social, and government policy *(e.g., fiscal and monetary policy)* trends; and possible actions of his competitors. Then, a list of all the relevant variables that have a bearing on the problem is

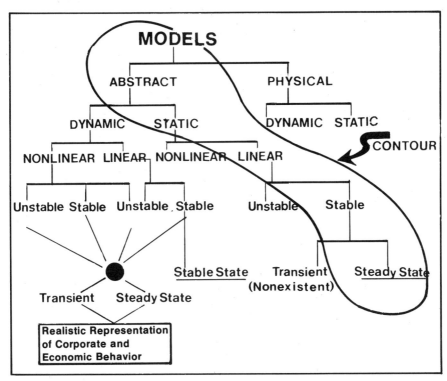

FIGURE 5.1   Classifications of models
SOURCE: Forrester (1961, p. 49)

compiled and divided into two sets: controllable and
non-controllable. One set consists of all those factors that are
under the control of the manager; while the second set consists of
those factors over which the manager has little control. A particular
combination of such controllable factors is termed a *strategy.* A
strategy is a course of action that the manager might employ in
order to achieve his objectives. A specific combination of
non-controllable factors, emerging as a result of random and
natural events, is called a *state of nature.*

The purpose of the *fourth* step is to state, in an explicit fashion,
the specific relationship among different variables and parameters
that are relevant to the problem. What emerges is a specific model.
The model could be a simple model that calls for optimization of a

"reward," "payoff," or "utility" as a function of controllable or non-controllable factors, such as

$$R = F(X_i, Y_j)$$

where

R = result, reward, or payoff measured in dollars, utility, or some other unit,

X_i = the set of controllable variables,

Y_j = the set of variables, and constants, which is not under the direct control of the manager, but which affects R, and

F = the functional relationship between the dependent variable R, and the independent variables X_i and Y_j.

The purpose of the *fifth* step is to formulate alternative strategies that could be employed to achieve objectives. The specific model, developed in step 4, can be used to generate strategies. Remember that we have defined the term strategy as a particular combination of controllable factors. The task of the manager here is to consider only those strategies that are feasible and viable in view of the available resources and specified constraints. The degree of detail with which the alternative strategies are specified is determined by the nature of the problem, pressures of time, and the hierarchical level at which the decision is being made. Further, the number of strategies could be finite or infinite, essentially depending upon whether the objective function or the utility function is assumed to be discrete or continuous.

The purpose of the *sixth* step is to project consequences of alternative strategies. Consequences of alternative strategies, or the payoffs associated with different strategies, are expressed in either monetary or utility terms. The mechanism through which such projections are made can vary from a sophisticated mathematical model to a simple intuitive prediction. At the very elementary level, especially where the number of finite strategies and the number of states of nature are very small, the consequences of alternative strategies may be predicted on an intuitive basis and shown in the form of payoff matrix as shown in Table 5.1.

The purpose of the *seventh* step is to choose the optimal strategy. This step requires that the optimal strategy be identified in accordance with a criterion of choice such as maximization of

TABLE 5.1

State of Nature

Strategy		N_1	N_2	N_3
	S_1	15	6	10
	S_2	3	4	16

profits or minimization of costs. If our criterion of choice is maximization, then we want to search for those values of X_i and Y_j that would give the maximum value of R.

The purpose of the *eighth* step is to implement the decision and maintain a system of control. This is the action step. Having identified the optimal strategy, the manager takes all the necessary steps to implement it. The question of follow-up and control, however, is of the utmost importance because the entire decision model is based on a set of assumptions including the assumption that the system is stable. If the optimal strategy is to remain optimal, a system of surveillance and control must be maintained to see whether any significant changes have taken place. If so, the circumstances would call for searching a new optimal strategy. Depending upon the specific formulation of the decision problem, the decision environment, or the predilections of the manager, some of the eight decision steps may be combined, or subsumed under different titles. But, they must be considered and executed—explicitly or implicitly, consciously or unconsciously.

Long-term care administrators are continually required to make important decisions regarding allocation of resources to patient care and related programs and in terms of their relationships with regulatory and rate-setting agencies. TAYLOR (Selection 14) discusses the implications of cognitive strain for decision-making effectiveness. Literature concerning the psychological processes of decision-makers, which underlie the operation of cognitive strain and which predispose them to the effects of cognitive strain, is reviewed. Next, the impact of cognitive strain on narrowly constraining or "bounding" rational decision-making is examined, and the choice strategies of satisficing and incrementalizing are criticized as failing to broaden the bounds of rational decision-making. Finally, elements of an eclectic choice strategy, designed to assist decision-makers in handling the informational demands of complex decision problems, are discussed.

While Taylor's article emphasized the psychological (behavioral) aspects of decision-making, EILON's article (Selection 15) deals with normative choice models. The decision process is described as a series of eight steps starting with information input and ending with decision "resolution" according to some "choice criteria" operating on the decision model. Various aspects of rationality in decision-making and the relationship of rationality to utility maximization are examined. It is emphasized that the most important aspects of the decision process are the model building and choice of criterion stages. A very important aspect of Eilon's article is that it treats explicitly the question of multiple objectives in decision-making. Eilon suggests the existence of a continuum of informal and formal procedures and the associated control consisting of a mix of "personalistic" and "impersonalistic" characteristics. It is pointed out that the type of control in decision-making is determined essentially by the degree of involvement of the decision-maker in various stages of the decision process. Control (formal or informal) and decision-making are related, and crucial points in the decision process are identified.

HERBERT SIMON's classic paper (Selection 16) is devoted to an examination of how organizational goals are formed. A distinction is made between goals and motives. Goals are defined as value premises that serve as inputs to decisions. Motives are any causes that lead individuals to select some goals rather than others as premises for their decisions. Organizational decision-making takes place in the context of multiple constraints or requirements, and sometimes one of these constraints is chosen as the goal of the action. However, for many purposes it is more meaningful to refer to the whole set of requirements as the (complex) goal of the action. Linear programming is employed to illustrate the relevance of multiple criteria in decision-making.

The author emphasizes the dual role of the goals of the action. First, the goals may be used directly to synthesize proposed solutions (alternative generation). Second, the goals may be used to test the satisfactoriness of a proposed solution (alternative testing). Goals can also be subdivided into *personal* and *role defined.* Personal goals motivate the individual to adopt the role, and then the goals and constraints appropriate to the role become a part of the decision-making system. Interpersonal differences in role behavior are described. An organizational decision-making system is described as one in which (1) particular decision-making processes are aimed at finding courses of action that are feasible or satisfactory in the light of multiple goals and constraints, and (2) decisions reached in one part of the organization enter as goals or constraints into the decisions being made in other parts of the organization. The author concludes that an organization goal is based on the constraints, or sets of constraints, imposed by the organizational roles, which have only indirect relation to the motives of the decision-makers.

14

Psychological Determinants of Bounded Rationality: Implications for Decision-Making Strategies

RONALD N. TAYLOR

INTRODUCTION

Since the mid-1950's when Herbert Simon first began to strew the seeds of behavioral decision-making among the orderly rows in the field of statistical decision theory, awareness of the severe limitations imposed upon rational decision-making by human cognitive ability has grown. Simon [75] and March and Simon [59] proposed that human decision-makers do exhibit rationality, but only within the constraints of their perception of a decision problem. Such constraints or boundaries typically have been found to be quite narrow when compared to the complexity of most organizational decision problems. Thus, while the capacity of humans tends to be overwhelmed by informational demands of these problems, Simon has suggested that decision-makers attempt to compensate for their limited abilities by constructing a simplified representation of the problem and behaving rationally within the constraints of this model. The notion of "bounded rationality," therefore, figures predominantly in theories of administrative decision-making as the basis for explaining departures from rationality (e.g., use of something other than a maximizing choice mode).

Bounded rationality frequently can be attributed to the operation of a

FROM: *Decision Sciences*, Vol. 6, July 1975, pp. 409-429.

psychological phenomenon which has been labeled "cognitive strain." Such a breakdown of a decision-maker's cognitive processes occurs when he is subjected to a state of information overload (i.e., when the informational demands of the decision environment exceed his information-processing capacity). Both experimental research in the laboratory and studies of actual organizations have demonstrated that the malady of cognitive strain is a chronic condition of administrative decision-making in governmental policy [50], military tactics [92], business [39], and natural resource management [38].

Such bounds placed upon rational decision-making can be viewed in the framework suggested by Reitman [70] as psychological constraints that can be either opened or closed as a decision problem is formulated for solution. In this sense, the decision-maker's limited ability to handle the information demands of a problem forces him to close many of the open constraints relevant to the problem; hence, he tends to formulate the problem in a restricted manner. Such restrictions frequently take the form of compensatory choice modes, two of which are examined below (i.e., satisficing and incrementalizing). These choice modes shield a decision-maker from cognitive strain by permitting him to formulate the problem in a simplistic manner, but both represent considerably less rationality in decision-making than many problems would warrant. By judiciously operating upon such psychological constraints, a decision-maker may more adequately formulate a problem by successively restructuring it. In the context of coping with bounded rationality, it seems appropriate to apply choice strategies which permit a decision-maker to optimize his information processing capacity and which enable him to expand the bounds within which rational decision-making can occur by not being forced to close out of hand so many constraints bounding the problem.

In the present paper we review the psychological bases of cognitive strain, examine the impact of such psychological characteristics on choice modes, and suggest ways in which the psychological constraints imposed by a decision-maker's cognitive limitations may be opened to increase the bounds of his rational decision-making. Our discussion of cognitive limitations on decision-making focuses on the individual decision maker, although it is apparent that many of these phenomena can be generalized to apply to groups and complex organizations (e.g., centrality in communication nets).

DETERMINANTS OF COGNITIVE STRAIN

As is evident from the above definition, cognitive strain represents an interaction of the characteristics of the decision-maker and his environmental characteristics. Although considerable attention has been addressed to the decision environmental influences on cognitive strain—MacCrimmon and Taylor [55], for example, examine the role of environmental complexity in terms of both multiplicity of factors and degree of interconnectedness among the factors on cognitive strain—relatively little attention has been given to the role of the decision-maker's psychological characteristics in predisposing him to cognitive strain.

While it is appropriate to describe the information load requirement of a decision problem as a single point, it is more suitable to view the information processing capacity of a decision-maker as having both upper and lower bounds of efficient information processing. Such a "band" of efficient information processing capacity is suggested by the Yerkes-Dodson law. This formulation, based on much empirical support, states that there is an optimal level of arousal for any task. The function relating quality of performance to level of arousal will have an inverted-U shape; performance will first improve, then deteriorate as arousal increases. Decision-makers, then, would be expected to perform best under conditions of intermediate levels of stress due to informational demands. At high levels of stress, relative to his information processing capacity, the dysfunctions of cognitive strain would occur.

Increasing information processing capacity should serve to shift the inverted-U shaped curve to the right so that more information can be processed at a given level of arousal. It should be kept in mind, however, that while such a strategy would expand the bounds of rational decision making, there still is an upper limit to information processing capacity. Hence, an optimal level of information load would exist for each decision-making environment. Greater information loads are not always better than lower loads. The upper limit of information load has received much theoretical discussion and its importance can be seen in the informational demands placed on air traffic controllers and on inspectors.

A lower limit of efficient information processing also exists. Remove informational demands, and the individual becomes bored and inattentive. Examples of the operation of a lower threshold of information load can be observed in vigilance difficulties noted for radar operators and gauge readers in automated plants or can be felt by anyone driving a freeway on a lonely night. For each decision-maker, then, a band of efficient information load exists, a band determined in part by his psychological characteristics. The wide individual differences observed in information processing capabilities are evident in performance on standardized tests used to select personnel for jobs requiring extremely high levels of information processing.

Bounds placed on rational decision-making by these forces can be relaxed by operating upon either the decision-maker or the decision environment or both to bring about correspondence between information load and processing capacity. For example, such strategies as "factoring into subproblems" and "aggregating information" represent attempts to reduce information load by modifying the decision environment. On the other hand, selecting decision-makers with high information processing capabilities or training them to overcome informational biases operates on the decision-maker to reduce cognitive strain. The choice strategies discussed below are those which seem appropriate to be used by a decision-maker without drastic structural changes in either the organization or his job (i.e., strategies that he may personally use to compensate for cognitive strain).

PSYCHOLOGICAL DETERMINANTS OF COGNITIVE STRAIN

Miller [63] found that humans were capable of retaining only about 7 chunks of information in short-term memory. A tendency for ability to recall information in a continuous short-term memory task to decline as storage load is increased (number of items that have not been tested for retention by the time a given item is recalled) has been well documented [25]. An explanation for the influence of short-term memory on information storage capacity has been advanced by Posner [67], and he suggests methods for combatting cognitive strain. He proposed that a decision-maker rarely stores a pure representation of information; rather, he is an active information handler who applies his knowledge of the nature of the information to reduce his memory load. A chess master, for example, appears able to store complex configurations of pieces on the chess board in his short-term memory as easily as a less expert player stores the position of a single piece. The concept of an "active" information processor is discussed further below as the basis for strategies to assist in aggregating information.

Psychological Attributes

Decision-makers differ sharply in ability to process information. Although empirical research in the psychological determinants of cognitive strain has been fragmentary, such research represents an essential basis for understanding why cognitive strain occurs and how it can be reduced. Among the psychological attributes of decision-makers which have been found to underlie information-processing capacity are intelligence, dogmatism, conceptual structure, risk-taking propensity and aspiration level.

In addition, researchers have examined related demographic attributes (e.g., age and experience) and behaviors manifested in decision-making (e.g., conservatism in opinion revision and pattern seeking) in searching for clues to the nature of cognitive strain. The research relating each of these decision-maker attributes to cognitive strain is briefly reviewed below.

Intelligence has generally been regarded as an important determinant of information-processing capacity. Thus, more intelligent decision-makers are better able to cope with high levels of information-processing load. Yet, research into this issue has led to quite mixed results regarding the impact of intelligence on decision processes [7] [68], perhaps due in part to different operational definitions of intelligence in these studies. In a study of managers, however, Taylor and Dunnette [89] observed that the more intelligent managers were able to handle information much more efficiently and diagnose information value more accurately than were less intelligent managers. On the basis of such evidence, it appears reasonable to conclude that intelligence is related to information-processing capacity although the nature of the relationship is far from clear. Further studies using measures of general mental ability and extending the investigation to include specific mental abilities (e.g., spatial visualization, computational skills) are badly needed.

One of the better-documented research findings is that *dogmatism* inhibits both pre-decisional and post-decisional information processing. Research using the Rokeach Dogmatism Scale [71] has shown that dogmatic decision-makers (i.e., those with closed belief systems) tend to make rapid decisions based upon relatively little information, and, once made, tend to hold those decisions confidently and inflexibly [7] [10]. On the basis of this line of research, Long and Ziller [51] have interpreted dogmatism as a defence mechanism that tends to inhibit information processing. Limiting information search closes the mind to new information and eliminates the need for the decision-maker to re-evaluate his self concept, a prospect he may find threatening. The dogmatic decision-maker would, therefore, be likely to unduly restrict his information input. The resulting reduction in his information processing capacity could serve as a severe constraint upon his rationality in making decisions, especially in decision problems which appear to threaten his self concept.

A decision-maker's susceptibility to cognitive strain is influenced by his *conceptual structure*. This aspect generally has been measured on a continuum of "abstractness" versus "concreteness". Concreteness is characterized by the use of a few dimensions of information and a simple integrating approach; abstractness refers to a tendency to process many dimensions of information and to use a complex approach to integration. Schroeder and Suedfeld [73] have found that abstract decision-makers are more information oriented and are able to process more information in complex decision environments. Concrete decision-makers, however, tend to experience cognitive strain at lower levels of environmental complexity and, hence, must restrict the amount of information they can process. Due to their ability to handle the cognitive demands for information search and integration, abstract decision-makers appear better prepared to cope with heavy informational demands. Also, their more efficient utilization of information, resulting from a tendency observed for them to "rescue" information for complex integrations, enables the abstract decision-maker to make decisions effectively under conditions of inadequate information base.

Propensity for taking risks is another psychological attribute of decision-makers that has been found to influence bounded rationality. The risky situation to which an individual high in this trait tends to expose himself involves both uncertainty about outcomes and the possibility of losses (including opportunity losses) of resources. A variety of measures of risk-taking propensity have been developed. These include psychological tests [2] [44], the mean-variance criterion [60], and the utility function [30] [56].

Bruner and his co-authors [12] have found that risk-taking propensity influences information-seeking strategies in concept formation problems. Two conjunctive strategies implying markedly divergent levels of risk are examined in their research—"conservative focusing" (finding one positive instance of the correct concept and varying one attribute at a time to identify the concept) and "focus gambling" (varying more than one attribute at a time). A decision-maker with a high risk-taking propensity would be expected to readily adopt the focus gambling strategy, thus permitting him to reduce the information demands in determining the correct concept. If, however, the individual using this strategy is not guided by the correct hunch, he may fail to attain the concept altogether.

These strategies appear to present the essence of risk-taking as a determinant of information processing capacity. Although a risky strategy may serve to reduce information load, it does so by exposing a decision-maker to potential losses because he does not fully utilize the information base. Taylor and Dunnette [89] have observed, however, that risk-prone decision-makers do not correspond to the popular stereotype of cavalier disregard for the information base in a willingness to expose themselves to risk. Rather, they were found to make relatively rapid decisions based on little information, but to process each item of information more slowly and judge its value for the decision more accurately than did risk-averse decision-makers.

The use of utility functions to assess risk-taking propensity has proved valuable to businessmen seeking to better understand their own and other's attitudes toward risk [31]. Although Spetzler [81] found a diversity of utility functions of the top managers within the same company, Swalm [87] found that most managers in a large company had very risk-averse utility functions. Rather than using the more risk neutral strategy that would be better for the company as a whole when small percentages of its resources were at stake, the managers seemed to be using their own very risk-averse utility. Having such knowledge provides the organization with a basis for encouraging managers at lower levels to take more risks.

A decision-maker's *level of aspiration* critically influences the bounds within which he can make rational decisions. It has been found to shape his effectiveness in problem identification, evaluation of decision alternatives, and setting negotiation bids. Aspiration level can be defined as a threshold that decision-makers attempt to attain [48] [74] in decision quality or productivity when making large numbers of decisions.

As examples of these two aspects of aspiration level, consider first a scientist striving to invent a product that will prove superior to all competing products of its type or an academician attempting to write the definitive article in his field. Here high aspiration level suggests that criteria against which inventions and articles are evaluated are stringent and that a decision-maker with this psychological characteristic would tend to expose himself to demanding information loads and subsequent cognitive strain in an effort to make the single decision. Alternatively, a production manager with high aspiration level may be confronted with a pressing array of decision problems and manifest his aspiration level by the sheer work load he undertakes. In so doing, we may expect him to be demanding of his information processing capabilities by undertaking a great range of decision problems, but to work to a moderate but acceptable standard in making each decision.

The bulk of research into aspiration level has dealt with productivity in decision tasks—the latter interpretation. It is instructive to examine some of the conditions which have been found to affect aspiration level in this sense: prior experiences of success or failure, setting specific goals, and receiving knowledge of results. The formulation generally used to specify the impact of aspiration level on task performance is Helson's *hypothesis of par*. This theory states that individuals set a standard of excellence for themselves which is usually beneath their capabilities and that they try to meet, but not exceed, this standard. In setting such standard, cognitive strain can be reduced by choosing an optimum level. Standards set too high lead to the frustration and dysfunctions of cognitive strain; standards set too low can be readily achieved, but such standards may not motivate sufficient information. Thus, a person may not be able to fully utilize his information-processing capability. Stedry [82] examines the implications of aspiration levels for setting tight vs. loose budgets, and

Ansoff [1] discusses the uses of aspiration level in corporate strategy decisions (e.g., setting goals such as achieving an increase of 20% in earnings per share).

The generally accepted conclusion from studies of prior success or failure and subsequent aspiration level is that successful performance leads to an increase in standards, while failure decreases standards set for future tasks [17] [18] [80]. While failure does not automatically lead to decreases in aspiration level or performance, the higher the ratio of success to failure the more stable the performance. Bourne [8] believed failure tended to reduce the individual's expectancy of success and led to less effort being expended or to less appropriate attempts at solution (e.g., looking for overly complex solutions). Perhaps, the latter interpretation operates, as Streufert suggested [85], because failure produced more integrative (strategically and pragmatically related) solutions.

Many experiments also have found that level of aspiration can be modified by arranging the task to suggest that high level of performance is expected. Mace [57], for example, improved performance in an aiming task simply by adding additional concentric rings within the established periphery, thus making what once appeared to be good performance look mediocre. The experimenters may also vary aspiration level by manipulating instructions to indicate that good scores have been obtained by others. Similarly, auctioneers are well aware that obtaining high prices on items sold early on raises the prices at which subsequent items are sold.

Much of the incentive which motivates the activities of a decision-maker comes from the consequences of his own actions. Research has shown that decision-makers tend to set more realistic standards and have a stronger motivation to resolve the problems they face when they are provided with knowledge of results concerning their performance relative to either their own previous performance or to the performance of others [83]. It seems clear that motivation to solve a problem can be enhanced by providing augmented feedback (i.e., from sources external to the decision-maker). This improvement is reflected in increased performance not only when the added feedback is present, but also when it is removed [79].

The effect of setting specific goals on motivation to resolve a problem has also been investigated and serves as the basis for the widely-used management by objectives programs. It is generally accepted that specific goals serve to motivate individuals with low task motivation to perform at higher levels. Bryan and Locke [13], for example, found that groups with specific goals were able to match the performance of initially more highly motivated groups who were told merely to "do your best." Bruckman and Campbell [11] provide additional findings concerning conditions affecting aspiration level for those interested in pursuing this topic further.

A demographic attribute of decision-makers that has been found instrumental in determining information-processing capacity is *age*. Age of decision-makers has frequently been said to contribute heavily to both the manner in which a decision is reached [41] [86] and decision quality [6] [91]. It would appear from the findings of these studies that older decision-makers are far more susceptible to the dysfunctional effects of information overload. Despite such findings from studies of decision-makers who are quite advanced in age and no longer in the work force, the implications of these studies for managerial decision-making depend upon the extent to which the impairments occur within the normal managerial age range.

Taylor [88] investigated age differences in information-processing ability for line managers with the influence of potentially contaminating variables (i.e., decision-making experience and management level) statistically removed. He found that the generally hypothesized sharp decline in information-processing capability did not emerge. Instead, it appears that the influence of age on information-processing behaviors is more complex than was previously believed. When the influence of decision-making experience and management level was held constant, older managers were found to be more accurate in judging information quality; however, they did require longer to reach decisions and were less confident and more flexible in holding the resulting decisions. Yet, age was not found to be significantly associated with decision quality, and the severe information-handling impairments suggested by some writers did not occur. Such evidence appears heartening for older decision-makers, possibly indicating that much of the impairments noted in earlier psychophysical studies were due to decline in perceptual ability with age, rather than decline in conceptual ability. Choice strategies to overcome perceptual limitations (e.g., acquire bi-focal glasses) would seem to be much easier to employ than strategies to compensate for impaired conceptual ability.

In an effort to tentatively map the relationships among psychological attributes that have been found instrumental in determining information-processing capability, Taylor and Dunnette [89] investigated the individual and joint contributions to decision processes of psychological and demographic attributes of decision-makers for a sample of 79 industrial managers. They concluded that the impact of cognitive attributes (e.g., intelligence, intellectual efficiency) on decision-making performance appears to be quite different from the effect of personality, interests and motivational attributes (e.g., dogmatism, risk-taking propensity, conceptual structure and interests).

Cognitive attributes contributed heavily to the judgmental aspects of decision-making of the type involved in cognitive strain. They appear to be important in judging the diagnosticity of information, retaining information in short-term memory, and aggregating both information and preferences for a decision. Cognitive attributes also were found to affect decision-making performance by influencing the capacity to process information. This hypothesis is indicated by the effects of intelligence on information processing rate and decision latency. These cognitive attributes seem, therefore, to have their greatest influence on information handling and choice behaviors, and to affect post-decisional processes rather minimally.

Personality, interests and motivational attributes were found to have their impact on the more stylistic or ideosyncratic decision-making behaviors (e.g., amount of information sought and processing rate) and were especially influential on post-decisional behaviors (e.g., decision confidence and decision flexibility in the face of adverse consequences of the choice). In a sequence of decisions, aspiration levels may possibly shift, producing corresponding changes in decision criteria or otherwise affecting the evaluative aspects of decision-making; but, this issue has not been systematically investigated.

Behavioral Phenomena

Considerable research has been addressed to psychological processes which can be inferred from information-processing and/or decision-making behavior. The implications of conclusions from this line of research are relevant to the issue of cognitive strain, although little attention has been given to investigating the extent to which decision-makers vary in exhibiting such phenomena. Two of these phenomena—pattern-seeking and conservatism—are examined here.

One of the more pervasive tendencies in human behavior is the search for meaning in stimulus patterns. Such phenomena have been labeled "Gestalt closure" and appear to be the basis for several perceptual biases observed in information processing. Because of the previously discussed limitations in human ability to process information, small numbers of concepts are typically used to classify information even when important information is suppressed in such broad categorizing [12]. Yet, Fillenbaum [29] found that individuals differ markedly in the width of categories they tend to use. Narrow categorizers would obtain more precise information, but impose considerably greater strain upon their ability to process information than would wide categorizers. Categorizing width is used below as the basis for several strategies to compensate for cognitive strain.

As further evidence that decision-makers tend to bias their perceptions in searching for meaning in information, Feldman [28] has found that people tend to assign patterns even when they know they are dealing with a random process. He has described the patterns that people insist they find in randomly generated sequences of binary digits. In a similar vein, some gamblers insist that sequences occur in spins of a roulette wheel, and the particular tendency to expect alternation (i.e., to think black is more likely if a sequence of reds has just appeared) is labelled the "gambler's fallacy."

Even people willing to accept the concept of random processes are subject to biases in the patterns they expect. For example, to most people the order of births of boys and girls, GBBGBG, seems more likely to occur than the sequence BBBGGG, since the former seems "more random." Similarly, in 6 tosses of a coin, only the sequence HTTHTH may appear really random. Kahneman and Tversky [36] discuss these and other fallacies.

Another perceptual bias noted in information-processing behavior is the extent to which such behavior departs systematically from the optimal Bayesian strategy [3]. The most pervasive deviation of this sort found in opinion revision is the tendency toward "conservativism". When exposed to additional information, decision-makers typically revise their posterior probability estimates in the direction specified by the optimal strategy, but the revision is often too small. The decision-makers act as though the data are less diagnostic than the Bayesian model would specify. In some studies [65] [66], the deviations were quite marked, sometimes requiring nine observations to revise judgments as much as the optimal strategy would specify for one observation. While several reasons for this bias have been suggested [24] and while some researchers [69] have concluded that the bias may be influenced as much by the measures that have been used (i.e., responses are not always systematically related to the Bayesian probabilities since they do not vary monotonically with the physical characteristics of the stimuli) as by the decision-maker's behavior, it does appear that such biases are real and that they influence the cognitive strain experienced by decision-makers. If one can assume a constant quality of decision, the inefficient use of information implied by the conservativism bias would necessitate considerably more information-processing activity.

SATISFICING AND INCREMENTALIZING AS COMPENSATORY CHOICE MODES

Two compensatory strategies have been widely discussed as representing typical decision-maker behavior in the face of complex decision problems—satisficing and incrementalizing. Because they are derived from observation of the behaviors of decision-makers attempting to cope with cognitive strain, these strategies are primarily descriptive. As prescriptive strategies, however, they possess inherent shortcomings. Although they recognize human limitations in information processing and may serve to shield a decision-maker from cognitive strain, they fail to enable him to expand the bounds of rationality in his decision-making efforts. They may be "good enough" for many administrative decisions, but offer little in the way of assistance to the decision-maker desiring to improve his performance.

The concept of a *satisficing* decision-maker has been suggested by Simon [75] as one strategy for reducing information-processing demands. In a satisficing choice mode, the decision-maker sets up a feasible aspiration level, then searches for alternatives until he finds one that achieves this level. As soon as a satisficing alternative is found, he terminates his search and selects that alternative. Studies have found that satisficing is commonly used by trust investment officers [16] and department store buyers [19].

Satisficing is primarily descriptive, but to the extent that a decision-maker cannot maximize, satisficing can be said to also possess some normative implications. Correspondence can be made between maximizing and satisficing at the formal level by considering satisficing as maximizing with a two-valued (i.e., satisfactory and unsatisfactory) utility function or by explicitly taking into account the costs of information search and by having an aspiration level that is based on costs and expectations in a direct utility assessment manner [15]. Yet, the major reason for proposing a "satisficing man" is that a decision-maker cannot make the required determinations for maximizing [54].

A satisficing strategy appears to represent an inappropriately simplistic perception of the typically complex administrative decision problems, but Cyert and March [19] point out that failure of local information search can lead the decision-maker to complex strategies. Although modification through trial and error learning may result in a complex search strategy, such a hit or miss procedure could be a costly experience.

Incrementalizing is an approach described by Lindblom [49] which relates quite closely to satisficing. In this strategy, a decision-maker makes successive limited comparison between existing programs or conditions and alternative courses of action. Few objectives are considered, and the alternatives are generally ones that are familiar to the decision-maker or that he can generate by local search. Potentially important outcomes, values, and alternative solutions are neglected, and agreement among decision-makers is sought instead of high goal attainment. Lindblom has labeled this approach "muddling through," and it forms the basis for the more formal strategy of disjointed incrementalism as proposed by Braybrooke and Lindblom [9]. Although the strategy has been suggested as a guide for decision-making in complex environments (e.g., making social policy decisions), it is primarily a descriptive model of how decisions are made.

EXPANDING THE BOUNDS OF RATIONALITY

Since decision-making performance is a joint function of psychological attributes of the decision-maker and environmental factors, rationality can be expanded by either 1) selecting and placing in decision making positions people who have the psychological prerequisites for "good" decision making or by 2) engineering the environment in such a way through problem formulation and diagnosis and information preference aggregation techniques that "better" decisions result. Our discussion of psychological attributes influential in determining cognitive strain may suggest criteria for selecting decision-makers, and the strategies presented below for coping with cognitive strain may be useful in designing programs to train decision makers. The second approach (engineering the decision environment) is emphasized here since it appears efficient in terms of organizational resources to offer strategies to assist existing managers.

The major shortcomings of satisficing and incrementalizing is that they serve only to reduce a decision-maker's perception of problem complexity; they do not permit him to optimize the bounds placed on rationality by his limited information-handling ability. An approach to specifying choice strategies that appears to have great potential for assisting decision-makers is one which draws upon an understanding of the psychological processes underlying cognitive strain to develop strategies for expanding information-processing capacity. Aspects of decision-making that seem to provide the greatest challenge to cognitive ability are: 1) problem formulation, 2) problem diagnosis, 3) information aggregation, and 4) preference aggregation. Accordingly, we review a range of techniques selected from several disciplines which appear to have merit for assisting a decision-maker to cope effectively with the information demands presented by each of these aspects.

While the discussion of these techniques and the selection of techniques for inclusion was necessarily abbreviated in the limited space available here, they should suggest additional techniques that a decision-maker may use. In developing a choice strategy to compensate for cognitive strain, a decision-maker is urged to explore the techniques available for dealing with each aspect of the problem and to eclectically choose a combination of techniques appropriate to the problem.

Reducing Cognitive Strain in Problem Formulation

As was mentioned in discussing compensatory choice modes, one common reaction of decision-makers to complex problems is to develop simplistic representations of the problem. Building meaningful models of complex systems is inherently difficult since attempts to make models too complex defeats the reason for building them. The challenge to a decision-maker is to develop a model which can be more easily manipulated than the complex system, yet which includes the key aspects of the system bearing upon the decision. Although almost any model represents something more complex than itself, a few models have been developed for dealing with complex systems. The two models discussed here use matrix representations to provide insights into the interrelationships of very complex systems such as those found in decision problems.

In dealing with complex decision environments, Simon [77] proposed that they be decomposed into the semi-independent components corresponding to their functional parts. Such a use of *decomposable matrices* is based on his view of complex systems as a hierarchy of levels in which the operation of the system at each level can be defined by describing its component functions. A good many decision environments meet the conditions specified for "nearly decomposable" systems—interactions among subsystems are weak but not negligible—and are appropriate for the application of this technique.

Nearly decomposable systems can be represented as hierarchies which reduce their complexity with relatively little loss of information. Since subparts belonging to different components of the system interact only weakly, the details of their interaction can be ignored. For example, while it is not necessary to observe in detail the interaction of each citizen of one country with each member of a second country in order to investigate the interface of the two countries, it would be advisable to examine the interactions among leaders of the two countries. By reducing the complexity of decision problems through ignoring related parts of a system's functional components, one is able to bring the informational requirements of the decision closer to the capabilities of human decision-makers.

An alternative approach for modelling complex decision problems involves application of *input-output models*, a technique developed by Leontieff [47] for macroeconomic planning. Such models have been widely used to analyze production and sales patterns, but they should be applicable to other complex administrative processes (e.g., modelling information flows). Input-output models systematically represent the interrelationships between the inputs and outputs of parts of a system such as an industry or an economy. While input-output formats have been presented as convenient ways to model complex environments in deterministic terms, one should remember that the model assumes a stable pattern of linear relationships between the various subsystems. The assumption of linearity makes it possible to manipulate a large system of variables and equations, and the ability to enlarge and refine the model without surpassing the limits of computational feasibility offsets any loss in accuracy due to representing non-linear relationships through linear equations. Since a major weakness of the input-output model is that a mistake in basic assumptions may render it useless for decision-making, it is advisable to provide such additional data as the sensitivity of the model to assumptions.

Reducing Cognitive Strain in Problem Diagnosis

Complex decision problems present special diagnostic difficulties. Clearly, the way a decision problem is defined can have considerable effect on the alternative solutions considered and the resources used in its solution [58]. Since a decision-maker is usually faced with multiple decision problems, he must be able to isolate sets of symptoms which are attributable to a common cause or causes and set priorities for attempting to solve the various problems confronting him. Simon [76] describes a common strategy for dealing with multiple problems in which a decision-maker sequentially shifts his attention from one problem to another. Thus, he permits the demands upon his attention to remain relatively light. Similarly, Drucker [22] has noted that managing for results in complex decision problems forces a decision-maker to set priorities for his solution attempts and to allocate his resources first to critical decisions.

Techniques discussed below to assist decision-makers in analyzing complex decision problems are: determining problem boundaries, analysis of changes, problem factoring, decomposing into controllable and uncontrollable elements, and means-end analyses of goals.

An approach for *determining boundaries* of complex problems has been specified by Kepner and Tregoe [40] in which the decision-maker attempts to determine the characteristics of the out-of-control part of the system and the characteristics of the in-control parts. Next, the decision-maker attempts to find single causes that will explain the part of the system that is out-of-control and differentiate it from the in-control part. Using this approach, one may compare units with low productivity with highly productive units to identify possible causes of low productivity. Characteristics common to all units (e.g., work methods or training programs) would be considered improbable causes of the production problem, and problem-solving efforts would be directed to characteristics which differ for high production and low production units (e.g., nature of equipment maintenance). Such an approach permits a decision-maker to keep in mind a good deal of information as he systematically bounds the problem.

Kepner and Tregoe [40] have also suggested that the many *changes* typically found in complex decision environments be systematically probed until the equilibrium-restoring action is found. Such an approach appears to be an efficient way to determine problem causes since problems generally result from a change in the decision situation (e.g., in materials, personnel, procedures). In the example above, changes that had occurred in the low productivity units prior to the time that productivity first began to fall would be examined.

Another strategy for dealing with complexity in decision problems is to classify the factors in the situation as either controllable or uncontrollable. Factors that are partially controllable can be decomposed into their controllable and uncontrollable components as suggested by Howard [35]. Since there is little use in attempting to solve a problem which is beyond the power of the decision-maker, such a strategy permits a person to focus on problems which he can potentially solve.

Information load requirements of complex decision problems can be reduced by *factoring the problem* into subproblems which in turn may be factored. Such an approach is a central feature of Braybrooke and Lindblom's disjointed incrementalism [9] and has been discussed by Koestler [43]. Breaking up a problem into subproblems is useful if there are only a few interrelationships among the subparts. If there are a number of interrelationships, the coordination problems would clearly outweigh the advantages of decomposition. Delegation of decision tasks is a common example of problem factoring. Factoring permits the use of specialization and division of labor when a decision-maker's subunits have differing capabilities and allows for parellelism in decision-making efforts.

A technique for reducing cognitive strain due to complex goal hierarchies or multiple goals is *means-end analysis* of a factored problem. This technique requires the decision-maker to compare the desired subgoal with the present state to find a solution that will move the present state closer to the goal. After the solution is applied, there may be a new gap to be reduced and new solutions to be considered. The General Problem Solver [64] is a computer program that has been constructed to operate on the basis of means-end analysis.

Reducing Cognitive Strain In Information Aggregation

Techniques for reducing the cognitive demands placed on the decision-maker as he aggregates information fall into several classes. He may be provided with a meaningful way to organize information (chunking); information may be appropriately arranged prior to his receiving it (aggregation level); his information search patterns may be specified (reliability index, risky search); or, he may be provided assistance in determining information diagnosticity (Probabilistic Information Processing System).

Chunking is a technique described by Simon [76] to assist a decision-maker in interpreting a complex array of stimuli by effectively organizing the information it contains. Information-processing capacity may be increased substantially by grouping the information into chunks or categories and ordering the categories in importance. For example, as he receives reports from operating units, a business executive may cognitively arrange the information they contain in terms of actual or anticipated decision problems. Perhaps, he may group the information pertaining to potential labor unrest, material shortages, etc. This process seems consistent with Posner's [67] concept of an active information handler, mentioned above, who uses his understanding of information available to him to reduce his memory load.

Marschak [60] has suggested a technique for efficiently aggregating information prior to its receipt by a decision-maker by partitioning it into the *optimal level of aggregation*. While detailed information (e.g., store-by-store sales) may be necessary for some decisions, a reduction in information load may be attained by the use of aggregated information (e.g., national sales). Aggregated information, however, should be used only where it is appropriate since it may be quite difficult to disaggregate information.

In making decisions requiring heavy information-processing demands, a decision-maker can reduce the amount of information he must process by selecting information from *relevant and reliable sources* and by ignoring information from other sources. Berlyne [4] theorized that decision-makers learn through implicit trial and error which sources or types of information can guide them to an optimal response by sequentially anticipating the outcomes of acting on each item. This procedure cannot be carried out in a random order [64]. Information sources can, however, be tried out in an order that reflects how successful each source has been in the past. This ordering reflects decision-maker biases, frequently only implied, towards information contributed by sources which have proven themselves reliable and relevant in his prior decisions. This phenomenon has been investigated in studies of impression formation [34] [72] and employment decisions [14], and it has been demonstrated that credence given to sources of information figures prominently in decision-making.

If a decision-maker is to use his prior experiences to reduce his information load, he may elect to make his evaluation of information sources explicit by attaching a value or weight to information from each source. Such an indexing scheme could also be extended to compensate for the frequently observed organizational phenomenon of uncertainty absorption—a tendency for uncertain or unreliable information to appear more certain and reliable as it is transmitted through the organizational hierarchy [93]. A reliability or certainty index would permit decision-makers at high levels in an organization to select information and weigh its importance judiciously; therefore, it would facilitate efficient information use.

The conjunctive strategies for information seeking described by Bruner and his colleagues [12] and briefly discussed above assist the decision-maker in reducing memory load by increasing the likelihood that the information he selects will be valuable and by regulating the level of risk he is willing to take. If a decision-maker has a hunch about the correct decision alternative, he can adopt a risky strategy (focus gambling) to reach a solution quickly and with less information processing. In the absence of such hunches, he would be advised to adopt a safe strategy (conservative focusing).

An illustration of the use of these strategies can be seen in new product introduction decisions. Potential products are conceptualized in terms of their characteristics or attributes, and marketers often think in terms of ideal levels for these attributes—i.e., those levels most desired by consumers. Test marketing is frequently used to determine these levels. If a range of products is to be tested sequentially to find the ideal levels, products differing from preceding semi-successful ones by a single attribute can be tested (focus gambling).

The *Probabilistic Information Processing System* (PIP) was introduced by Edwards and his associates [23] [24] as a technique to assist decision-makers in compensating for conservatism and other inefficiencies in human information processing. It is a system in which a decision-maker estimates likelihood ratios, and a computer aggregates these across data and across hypotheses according to Bayes' theorem. The PIP system has been used in a variety of military problems [37] and has been proposed for use in medicine [32] [52] and in probation decisions [61].

By reducing the decision-makers' computational demands, the PIP system improves both speed and accuracy of decision-making in complex environments. Its advantages include the capacity to screen information for relevance, to filter out noise, to apply appropriate weight to each information element, and to specify an optimal procedure for extracting all the certainty available in the information.

Reducing Cognitive Strain in Preference Aggregation

The challenge presented to a decision-maker's cognitive ability by complex decision problems frequently results from a multitude of attributes or factors to consider. Three strategies that appear particularly well suited to assisting the decision-maker to compensate for cognitive strain are a method of sequential elimination of decision altenatives (specification of constraints), a weighting method (bootstrapping with regression), and a mathematical programming method (interactive programming). Readers interested in a more thorough treatment of multiple objective decision-making techniques are referred to an excellent review by MacCrimmon [53].

One of the least demanding techniques for multiple attribute decision making is for the decision maker to *specify preference constraints* and to satisfice by attempting to find a decision alternative that just meets, but not necessarily surpasses, the constraints [20] [18]. A constraint for graduate school admission decisions may be "applicants must have an undergraduate degree from an accredited school." A number of such constraints can be specified to operate either disjunctively (i.e., only one constraint need be met) or conjunctively (all constraints must be met). This simple technique has been widely used by consumers, bank trust investment officers, personnel specialists and psychiatric counselors [5] [16] [42] [78].

When each decision is quite complex, but requires a number of similar decisions to be made, cognitive strain can frequently be reduced by applying a *linear regression model* of a decision maker's behavior. Such models have been developed for employment decisions, diagnosis of X-rays, admission of graduate students, deciding on workmen's compensation awards, and a host of other decisions [21] [33] [45]. In an employment decision, for example, factors describing job candidates (e.g., employment history, psychological test scores) can be used to predict success on the job. If the fit of the linear equation is good, then, this equation can be used in future employment decisions for preliminary screening of job applicants. The reduction in the number of job applicants to consider resulting from this weeding out of clearly unsuccessful applicants would bring the informational demands of the decision closer to the capabilities of a decision-maker.

An intriguing finding of investigations into the use of bootstrapping with linear models is that the linear model can frequently do better than the decision-maker for whose preferences it is a paramorphic representation. The reasons for this are unclear, but it appears that the model may smooth out the choices and avoid the unsystematic shifting of attention that sometimes misleads the human decision-maker [21]. Kunreuther [46] describes conditions under which one should rely on a simple model in production planning and under which the decision-maker would be advised to contravene it. This issue has also been examined by Meehl [62] in the context of psychiatric diagnosis. He concluded that in the absence of strong additional evidence which would invalidate the linear regression prediction, a decision-maker can make better decisions by relying on the model rather than on his "clinical" judgment.

Finally, when the available alternatives can be defined by mathematical constraints and the decision problem has more of a design than a simple choice orientation, *interactive programming* can be used to reduce cognitive strain. One application of this technique is in scheduling an academic department [27]. This procedure is relatively undemanding of the decision-maker's cognitive ability since it requires him only to identify a feasible alternative, then trade off incremental changes in attribute values from this reference point. These trade-offs become part of an objective function in a mathematical programming problem, and a new solution is obtained. The technique continues in an iterative manner using the decision-maker to make local trade-off inputs, but leaving all calculations up to a computer algorithm.

A CONCLUDING NOTE

The central role of cognitive strain in decision-making is the focus of this paper. A wealth of literature relevant to the causes of cognitive strain, the dynamics of its operation, and ways to overcome its adverse consequences has been developed by several disciplines; yet, little effort has been given to systematically relating the themes drawn from this literature. Hopefully, the approach taken here will enhance appreciation of both the pervasiveness of cognitive strain in administrative decision-making and the severe limitations it places upon the ability of a decision-maker to formulate problems, to diagnose them accurately, and to perform the computational and aggregative processes required in reaching sound decisions. An additional motive for this paper was normative, that is, to suggest techniques that may prove helpful to decision-makers who experience the dysfunctions of cognitive strain. Finally, it is hoped that by integrating theories, research conclusions, and methods from various disciplines into a common view of this phenomenon, it may be possible to highlight common interests and promote interdisciplinary research.

REFERENCES

[1] Ansoff, H.I. *Corporate Strategy*. New York: McGraw-Hill, 1965.
[2] Atkinson, J.W. "Motivational Determinants of Risk-Taking Behavior." *Psychological Review*, Vol. 64 (1957), pp. 359-372.
[3] Bayes, T. "Essay Towards Solving a Problem in the Doctrine of Chances." *The Philosophical Transactions*, Vol. 53, 1963, pp. 370-418.

[4] Berlyne, D.E. *Conflict, Arousal and Curiosity.* New York: McGraw-Hill, 1960.

[5] Bettman, J.R. "The Structure of Consumer Choice Process." *Journal of Marketing Research,* Vol. 8 (1971), pp. 465-471.

[6] Birren, J.C., A. Jerome, and F. Chown. "Age and Decision Strategies." in A.T. Welford, ed., *Interdisciplinary Topics in Gerontology,* Vol. IV. 1961, pp. 23-26.

[7] Block, J. and P. Petersen. "Some Personality Correlates of Confidence, Caution, and Speed in a Decision Situation." *Journal of Abnormal Social Psychology,* Vol. 51 (1955), pp. 34-41.

[8] Bourne, L.E. Jr., B.R. Ekstrand, and R.C. Dominowski. *The Psychology of Thinking.* Englewood Cliffs, N.J.: Prentice-Hall, 1971.

[9] Braybrooke, D., and C.E. Lindbolm. *A Strategy of Decision.* New York: Free Press, 1963.

[10] Brengelmann, J.C. "Abnormal and Personality Correlates of Certainty." *Journal Mental Science,* Vol. 105 (1959), pp. 142-162.

[11] Bruckman, P. and D.T. Campbell. "Hedonic Relativism and Planning the Good Society." in M.H. Appley, ed., *Adaptation-Level Theory: A Symposium.* New York: Academic Press, 1971.

[12] Bruner, J.S., J.J. Goodnow, and G.A. Austin. *A Study of Thinking.* New York: Science Editions, Inc., 1956.

[13] Bryan, J.F. and E.A. Locke. "Goal Setting As a Means For Increasing Motivation." *Journal of Applied Psychology,* Vol. 53 (1967), pp. 274-277.

[14] Carlson, R.E. "Selection Interview Decisions: The Relative Influence of Appearance and Factual Written Information on an Interviewer's Final Rating." *Journal of Applied Psychology,* Vol. 51 (1967), pp. 461-468.

[15] Charnes, A. and W.W. Cooper. "Deterministic Equivalents for Optimizing and Satisficing Under Change Constraints." *Operations Research,* Vol. 11 (1963), pp. 18-39.

[16] Clarkson, G.P.E. *Portfolio Selection: A Simulation of Trust Investment,* Englewood Cliffs, N.J.: Prentice-Hall, 1962.

[17] Cofer, C.N. and M.H. Appley. *Motivation: Theory and Research.* New York: Wiley, 1961.

[18] Coombs, C.H. *A Theory of Data.* New York: Wiley, 1964.

[19] Cyert, R.M. and J.G. March. *A Behavioral Theory of the Firm.* Englewood Cliffs, N.J.: Prentice-Hall, Inc., 1963.

[20] Dawes, R. "Social Selection Based on Multidimensional Criteria." *Journal of Abnormal Psychology,* Vol. 23 (1964), pp. 104-109.

[21] Dawes, R. "Graduate Admissions: A Case Study." *The American Psychologist,* 1971.

[22] Drucker, P.F. "Managing for Business Effectiveness." *Harvard Business Review,* Vol. 41 (1963), pp. 53-60.

[23] Edwards, W. "Man and Computers." *Psychological Principles in System Development,* R.M. Gangne, ed. New York: Holt, Rinehart & Winston, 1962, pp. 75-114.

[24] Edwards, W. "Conservatism in Human Information Processing." *Formal*

Representation of Human Judgment, B. Kleinmuntz, ed. New York: John Wiley and Sons, 1968.

[25] Elmes, D.G. "Short-Term Memory as a Function of Storage Load," *Journal of Experimental Psychology*, Vol. 81 (1969), pp. 203-204.

[26] Feather, N.T. "Effects of Prior Success and Failure on Expectations of Success and Subsequent Performance." *Journal of Personality and Social Psychology*, Vol. 3 (1966), pp. 287-298.

[27] Feinberg, A. *An Experimental Investigation of an Interactive Approach For Multi-Criterion Optimization With An Application to Academic Resource Allocation*, unpublished Ph.D. dissertation, UCLA, 1972.

[28] Feldman, J. "Simulation of Behavior in the Binary Choice Experiments." In E.A. Feigenbaum and J. Feldman, eds. *Computer and Thought.* New York: McGraw-Hill, 1963, pp. 329-346.

[29] Fillenbaum, S. "Some Stylistic Aspects of Categorizing Behavior." *Journal of Personality*, Vol. 27 (1959).

[30] Friedman, M. and L.J. Savage. "The Utility Analysis of Choices Involving Risk." *Journal of Political Economics*, Vol. 56 (1948), pp. 279-304.

[31] Grayson, C.J. *Decisions Under Uncertainty*, Boston: Harvard University Press, 1960.

[32] Gustafson, D.H. "Evaluation of Probabilistic Information Processing in Medical Decision Making." *Organizational Behavior and Human Performance*, Vol. 4, pp. 20-34.

[33] Hoffman, P.J., P. Slovic, and L.G. Rorer. "An Analysis-of-Variance Model for the Assessment of Configural Cue Utilization in Clinical Judgment." *Psychological Bulletin*, Vol. 68 (1968), pp. 338-349.

[34] Hovland, C.I. "Effects of the Mass Media of Communication." *Handbook of Social Psychology*, G. Lindzey, ed. Cambridge: Addison-Wesley, 1954.

[35] Howard, R.A. "Proximal Decision Analysis." *Management Science*, Vol. 17 (1971), pp. 507-541.

[36] Kahneman, D. and A. Tversky. "Subjective Probability: A Judgment of Representativeness," *Oregon Research Institute Bulletin*, Vol. 10 (1970).

[37] Kaplan, R.J. and J.R. Newman. "Studies in Probabilistic Information Processing." IEEE Transaction, HFE-7, 1966, pp. 49-63.

[38] Kates, R.W. *Hazard and Choice Perception in Flood Plain Management* Chicago: University of Chicago, Dept. of Geography, 1962.

[39] Katona, G. *Psychological Analysis of Economic Behavior.* New York: McGraw-Hill, 1951.

[40] Kepner, C.H. and B.B. Tregoe. *The Rational Manager.* New York: McGraw-Hill, 1965.

[41] Kirchner, W.K. "Age Differences in Short-Term Retention of Rapidly Changing Information." *Journal of Experimental Psychology*, Vol. 55 (1958), pp. 352-358.

[42] Kleinmuntz, B. "The Processing of Clinical Information by Man and Machine." *Formal Representation of Human Judgment*, B. Kleinmuntz, ed. New York: John Wiley and Sons, 1968.

[43] Koestler, A. *The Ghost in the Machine.* London: Hutchinson Publishing Group, Ltd., 1967.

[44] Kogan, N. and M.A. Wallach. *Risk-Taking: A Study in Cognition and Personality.* New York: Holt, Rinehart and Winston, 1964.

[45] Kort, F. "A Non Linear Model for the Analysis of Judicial Decisions." *The American Political Science Review,* Vol. 62 (1968), pp. 546-555.

[46] Kunreuther, H. "Extensions of Bowman's Theory on Managerial Decision-Making" Management Science, Vol. 15 (1969), pp. 415-439.

[47] Leontief, W. *Input-Output Economics.* Oxford: Oxford University Press, 1966.

[48] Lewin, K., L. Dembo, L. Festinger, and P. Sears. "Level of Aspiration." *Personality and Behavior Disorders.* J.M. Hunt, ed. New York: Ronald Press, 1944.

[49] Lindblom, C.E. "The Science of Muddling Through." *Public Administration Review,* Vol. 19 (1959), pp. 79-88.

[50] Lindblom, C.E. *The Intelligence of Democracy: Decision Making Through Mutual Adjustment.* New York: Free Press, 1965.

[51] Long, Barbara H. and R.C. Ziller. "Dogmatism and Predecisional Information Search." *Journal of Applied Psychology,* Vol. 49 (1965), pp. 376-378.

[52] Lusted, L.B. *Introduction to Medical Decision Making,* Springfield, Illinois: Thomas, 1968.

[53] MacCrimmon, K.R. "An Overview of Multiple Objective Decision Making." In *Multiple Criterion Decision Making,* J.L. Cochrane and M. Zeleny, eds. University of South Carolina Press, 1973.

[54] MacCrimmon, K.R. "Descriptive and Normative Implications of the Decision Theory Postulates." In *Risk and Uncertainty,* K. Borch and J. Mossin eds. London: Macmillan, 1968.

[55] MacCrimmon, K.R. and R.N. Taylor. "Decision-Making and Problem-Solving." In *Handbook of Industrial and Organizational Psychology,* M.D. Dunnette ed. Rand-McNally, in press.

[56] MacCrimmon, K.R., and M. Toda. "The Experimental Determination of Indifference Curves." *Review of Economic Studies,* Vol. No. 4 (1969), pp. 433-445.

[57] Mace, C.A. *Incentives: Some Experimental Studies.* London: Industrial Health Research Board, 1935.

[58] Maier, N.R.F. "Reasoning in Humans, II. The Solution of a Problem and its Appearance in Consciousness." *Journal of Comparative Psychology,* Vol. 13 (1931), pp. 181-194.

[59] March, J.G. and H.A. Simon. *Organizations.* New York: Wiley, 1958.

[60] Markowitz, H. *Portfolio Selection.* New York: Wiley, 1959.

[61] McEachern, A.W. and J.R. Newman. "A System for Computer-Aided Probation Decision-Making." *Journal for Research on Crime and Delinquency,* (July, 1969).

[62] Meehl, P.E., *Clinical vs. Statistical Prediction,* University of Minnesota, Minneapolis, 1954.

[63] Miller, G.A. "The Magical Number Seven, Plus or Minus Two: Some Limits on Our Capacity for Processing Information." *Psychological Review,* Vol. 63 (1956), pp. 81-97.

[64] Newell, A., J.C. Shaw, and H.A. Simon. "Report on a General Problem-

Solving Program." *Proceedings of the International Conference on Information Processing.* Paris: UNESCO, 1960.

[65] Peterson, C.R. and A.J. Miller. "Sensitivity of Subjective Probability Revision." *Journal of Experimental Psychology,* Vol. 70 (1965), pp. 526-533.

[66] Phillips, L.D. and W. Edwards. "Conservatism in a Simple Probability Inference Task." *Journal of Experimental Psychology,* Vol. 72 (196), pp. 346-354.

[67] Posner, M.I. "Immediate Memory in Sequential Task." *Psychological Bulletin,* Vol. 60 (1963), pp. 346-354.

[68] Pruitt, D.G. "Informational Requirements in Making Decisions." *American Journal of Psychology,* Vol. 74 (1961), pp. 433-439.

[69] Rapoport, A., and T.S. Wallsten. "Individual Decision Behavior." *Annual Review of Psychology,* (1972), pp. 131-176.

[70] Reitman, W.R. "Heuristic Decision Procedures, Open Constraints, and the Structure of Ill-defined Problems." *Human Judgments and Optimality,* M. Shelley and G. Bryan, eds. New York: Wiley, 1964.

[71] Rokeach, M. *The Open and Closed Mind.* New York: Basic Books, 1960.

[72] Rosenbaum, M.E. "The Source of Information in Impression Formation." *Psychological Science,* Vol. 8 (1967), pp. 175-176.

[73] Schroeder, H.M. and P. Suedfeld. *Personality Theory and Information Processing.* New York: Ronald Press, 1971.

[74] Siegel, S. "Level of Aspiration and Decision Making." *Psychological Review,* Vol. 64 (1957), pp. 253-262.

[75] Simon, H.A. *Administration Behavior,* (2nd ed.). New York: Macmillan Company, 1957.

[76] Simon, H.A. *The New Science of Management Decision.* New York: New York University, 1960.

[77[Simon, H.A. *The Science of the Artificial.* Cambridge, Mass.: The M.I.T. Press, 1969.

[78] Smith, R.D. and P.S. Greenlaw. "Simulation of a Psychological Decision Process in Personnel Selection." *Management Science,* Vol. 13 (1967), B-409-B-419.

[79] Smode, A. "Learning and Performance in a Tracking Task Under Two Levels of Achievement Information Feedback." *Journal of Experimental Psychology,* Vol. 56 (1958), pp. 297-304.

[80] Stolley, C.M. and R. Stagner. "Effects of Magnitude of Temporal Barriers, Type of Goal and Perception of Self." *Journal of Experimental Psychology,* Vol. 51 (1956), pp. 62-70.

[81] Spetzler, C.S. "The Development of a Corporate Risk Policy for Capital Investment Decisions." *IEEE Transactions of Systems Science and Cybernetics,* Vol. SSC-4 (1968), pp. 279-300.

[82] Stedry, A.C. *Budget Control and Cost Behavior.* Englewood Cliffs, N.J.: Prentice-Hall, 1960.

[83] Steers, R.M. and L.W. Porter. "The Role of Task-Goal Attributes in Employee Performance." *Psychological Bulletin,* Vol. 81 (1974), pp. 434-452.

[84] Streufert, S. and C.H. Castore. "Effects of Increasing Success and Failure on Perceived Information Quality." *Psychonomic Science,* Vol. 11 (1968), pp. 63-64.

[85] Streuffert, S., P. Suedfeld, and M. Driver. "Conceptual Structure, Information Search and Information Utilization." *Journal of Personality and Social Psychology*, Vol. 2 (1965), pp. 736-740.

[86] Surwillo, W.W. "The Relation of Decision Time to Brain Wave Frequency and to Age." *Electroencephalographic Clinical Neurophsialogy*, Vol. 16 (1964), pp. 510-514.

[87] Swalm, R.O. "Utility Theory—Insights into Risk Taking." *Harvard Business Review*, Vol. 44 (1966), p. 123.

[88] Taylor, R.N. "Age and Experience as Determinants of Managerial Information—Processing and Decision-Making Performance." *Academy of Management Journal*, Vol. 18 (1975), pp. 74-81.

[89] Taylor, R.M. and M.D. Dunnette. "Influence of Dogmatism, Risk-Taking Propensity and Intelligence on Decision-Making Strategies of a Sample of Industrial Managers." *Journal of Applied Psychology*, Vol. 59 (1974), pp. 420-423.

[90] Taylor, R.N. and M.D. Dunnette. "Relative Contribution of Decision-Maker Attributes to Decision Processes." *Organizational Behavior and Human Performance*, Vol. 12 (1974) pp. 286-298.

[91] Weir, M.W. "Developmental Changes in Problem Solving Strategies." *Psychological Review*, Vol. 71 (1964), pp. 473-490.

[92] Wholstetter, R. *Pearl Harbor: Warning and Decision*. Stanford, California: Stanford University Press, 1962.

[93] Woods, D.H. "Improving Estimates that Involve Uncertainty." *Harvard Business Review*, Vol. 44 (1966), pp. 91-98.

[94] Ziller, R.L. "A Measure of the Gambling Response Set in Objective Tests." *Psychometrika*, Vol. 22 (1957), pp. 289-292.

15

What Is A Decision?

SAMUEL EILON

DEFINITIONS

An examination of the literature reveals the somewhat perplexing fact that most books on management and decision theory do not contain a specific definition of what is meant by a *decision*. One can find detailed descriptions of decision trees, discussions of game theory and analyses of various statistical treatments of payoffs matrices under conditions of uncertainty, but the definition of the decision activity itself is often taken for granted and is associated with making a choice between alternative courses of action. As Fishburn puts it:

> Solving the decision model consists of finding a strategy for action the expected relative value of which is at least as great as the expected relative value of any other strategy in a specified set. The prescriptive criterion of a strategy will be maximization of the decision maker's total expected relative value. [3, p. 11]

A concise description of alternative definitions of a decision is given by Ofstad, who says:

> To say that a person has made a decision may mean (1) that he has started a series of behavioral reactions in favor of something, or it may mean (2) that he has made up his mind to *do* a certain action, which he has no doubts

FROM: *Management Science*, Vol. 16, December 1969, pp. B172-B189.

that he ought to do. But perhaps the most common use of the term is this: 'to make a decision' means (3) to make a judgment regarding what one *ought* to do in a certain situation after having deliberated on some alternative courses of action. [4, p. 15]

He then adds that (3) has the support of philosophical tradition. To quote Churchman,

"The manager is the man who decides among alternative choices. He must decide which choice he believes will lead to a certain desired objective or set of objectives." [1, p. 17]

The essential ingredients in this definition are that the decision-maker has *several alternatives* and that his choice involves a *comparison* between these alternatives and the *evaluation of their outcomes*.

THE DECISION PROCESS

But before we concentrate on the final selection of a course of action, it is necessary to consider the decision activity as a whole. What are the mental processes that the decision maker goes through before he arrives at his conclusion?

Figure 1 is an attempt to describe the decision process in a schematic form: First, there is an information input, say from some data processing machinery. This is followed by an analysis of the information material with the purpose of ascertaining its validity and discriminating between its significant and insignificant parts. The analysis leads to the specification of performance measures, which provide the basis for determining how a particular course of action is to be judged, and then to the construction of a model in order to describe the behaviour of the system for which the manager is asked to make a decision.

In a production-marketing system, for example, the measures of performance may include profit, mean level and/or variance of plant utilization, level of meeting customer demand, and so on. Thus, and given courses of action, whether they represent existing policies or whether they are hypothetical propositions for new policies, can be described by arrays of the measures of performance that are thought to be most relevant.

A set of alternatives (or "strategies" in the language of the theory of games) is enumerated and predictions are then made regarding the possible outcomes of each alternative. In order to be able to select between them, a criterion for comparing outcomes in the light of their respective measures of performance is set up and finally the selection (called here *resolution*) is made.

There are several comments that should be made here. First, the term *decision* is identified in many people's minds with what is called here

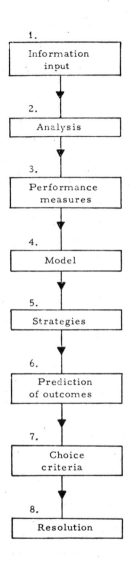

1.
Information
input

2.
Analysis

3.
Performance
measures

4.
Model

5.
Strategies

6.
Prediction
of outcomes

7.
Choice
criteria

8.
Resolution

FIGURE 1. The decision process

resolution, while some would argue that a decision includes the determination of selection criteria as well. Most students of statistical decision theory insist that the prediction of outcomes of events is an indispensable part of the decision activity, and some suggest that the enumeration of strategies is also an integral component of decision-making. It will become clear from the following discussion, I hope, that the various steps in the decision process are so interrelated and that each may have such significant implications for others, that it is essential to examine all these steps in order to identify the crucial links in the chain of events that leads to the final selection of a particular course of action.

Secondly, there is a need to distinguish between *rational* and *irrational* resolution. Dictionary definitions of the term *rational* ("endowed with reason, sensible, sane, moderate", etc.) are not entirely adequate for our purposes. Churchman discusses the concept of reason at some length and comments that

> perhaps the most predominant in the history of thought has been a definition of reason that has tied it closely to logic. The general idea here is that reason consists of logical and consistent steps that go from first principles to rigidly derived conclusions. The steps satisfy all the requirements that formal logic imposes on the so-called reasoning process. [1, p. 95]

Churchman is not satisfied with this concept and strongly suggests that "rationality has to do with goals as well as the means of the attainment of goals" [1, p. 102] and disagrees with those to whom "it will seem futile to ascribe rationality to goals, unless the goals are regarded as intermediate means to further goals," [1, p. 121]. The implication of Churchman's arguments is that questions of ethics and morality cannot be divorced from the concept of rationality, since they are often embedded in the determination of goals, otherwise we can never tell "what is absolutely right." The proposition that rationality should be judged in terms of what an individual wishes to attain, that if his intentions are good he is rational and if they are evil he is irrational, is of course contentious. For the sake of our discussion, however, I propose a more restricted definition of rational behaviour. What I mean by rational resolution is that the decision-maker conforms to the selection criterion, namely that if after applying the criterion a course of action A is shown to superior to B, the decision-maker does in fact select A in preference to B. If he does not, then the resolution is *irrational*. Further aspects of rationality in decision-making are discussed later.

Thirdly, if the discussion of the decision-making process is confined to rational decisions, it follows that every step in the process described in Figure 1 is indispensable and that the steps must proceed in the order specified: Information is essential for analysis and for defining measures of performance; without these preliminaries, no model building related to the real world is possible, and without a model to describe the behaviour of the system that the decision maker is trying to control, no alternative courses of action (or strategies) can be considered; the prediction of outcomes is meaningless unless it corresponds to a set of alternative strategies, and the method for choosing between them may well have to be delayed until the expected outcomes have been listed. The final act, that of resolution, is specified by the criterion of choice.

Each step in this process has as its input the outcome of activities in preceding steps and in turn it provides an input to the next step. The use that is made of these inputs varies from step to step: All the relevant information, for example, is useful for analysis and for model building, but all the detailed data are rarely needed to define performance measures, and once the model has been constructed it embodies the previous steps to an extent that many information details may be ignored in subsequent steps.

Fourthly, it should be noted that while—for the sake of simplicity—the decision process is depicted in Figure 1 as a chain of sequential activities, it very often takes the form of recurrent chains with feedback. Figure 2 described in schematic form the model building process with feedback. Model building is very similar to proposing a hypothesis in the hypothetico-deductive scientific method. The model describes the interrelationships between variables in the system; it attempts to show cause and effect; in short, it is designed to provide a predictive tool, so that the controller of the system can proceed to manipulate the variables under his control in order to achieve some desired objectives. But in structuring a theory any given hypothesis needs to be tested and scrutinised, through the design of new experiments and the collection of fresh information, and a model constructed as a part of the decision process must be examined in very much the same way. At any stage in this process questions may arise as to the validity of the information, the adequacy of the analysis, the meaning of performance measures, the need for fresh evidence to test the model and some of its implications. This recurrent procedure permeates throughout the decision process.

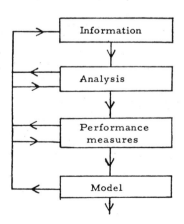

FIGURE 2. Model building with feed-back

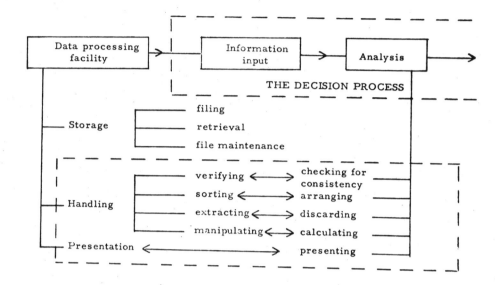

FIGURE 3. Data processing and analysis

HOW DATA PROCESSING IMPINGES ON ANALYSIS

The decision process starts with an information input and it is often asserted that information processing that precedes this input is quite distinct from the subsequent analysis that marks the beginning of the decision process proper.

If we examine, however, the activities that are involved in data or information processing on the one hand and in analysis on the other, we find that the line of demarcation is far from being distinct, if it can be drawn at all. Data processing consists of three major activities [2]: data and information stage, data handling and the presentation of information, and these activities may be further divided into several categories, as shown in Figure 3.

Let us now turn to analysis. What does the decision-maker do when he is engaged in analysis? First, he checks for consistency of the data that he is presented with, and if he detects inconsistencies, he demands an explanation. This activity of *checking for consistency* is not very different from *verifying*, which is part of data handling. Secondly, he arranges the information in a certain sequence and in a form that allows him and his colleagues to comprehend the full import of the information, and this activity of *arranging* is very similar to *sorting* in data handling.

The decision-maker then discards that information which he considers to be less significant for his analysis than the information that he chooses to retain for further examination, and this is precisely what *extracting* in data handling is designed to do. He then carried out *calculations*, which are akin to *data manipulating* in data handling, and finally he presents the results in a form that is most convenient and useful for the model building stage.

All these activities, that form a part of what I call "analysis" (namely, checking data to eliminate inconsistencies, arranging data, discriminating between more significant and less significant information, computing new sets of data and finally summarising and presenting the results), are precisely mirrored by those listed under the heading "data processing" (except for data storage). Data processing is, therefore, not distinct from analysis and the two greatly overlap.

In fact, if the decision-maker were clearly to specify in advance how the information should be handled prior to presentation, then the whole function of analysis could be transferred to the data processing facility, so that information input to the decision-maker is then already presented in a digested and convenient form for him to proceed immediately to the next stages in the decision process, namely to determining performance measures and to constructing a model.

In reality, of course, there are many circumstances in which the whole function of analysis cannot be transferred in this way. First, we find that many decision makers loathe delegating this function and thereby allowing the data processing facility to encroach on their domain of responsibility. Secondly, and this is perhaps fundamentally more important, the decision-maker is not always in a position to specify in advance what analysis should be undertaken. As already intimated in the diagram in Figure 2, analysis, setting performance measures and model building, are parts of an iterative process. Very often, it is only after an attempt has been made to construct a model and after its weaknesses have been exposed, that the need for further analysis can be realised and a re-evaluation of the specified performance measures can be undertaken.

There is, therefore, a limit to the degree of transfer of the analysis function from the decision-maker to the data processing facility, even when the decision-maker genuinely acquiesces in such a move. However, the point is worth making that when model building processes are comparatively routine with few novel features—and administration in industry and government abounds with such instances—a remarkable slice of the analysis function *can* be transferred from the decision process to data processing and there is a great deal of evidence to suggest that this transfer is accelerated when the data processing facility takes the form of a computer-based information centre.

What must be realised is that even when the computer centre assumes an increasingly important role in the analysis function, the decision-maker must retain the responsibility for drawing specifications for the output of the computer centre, not just to ensure that this output is relevant to the subsequent model building stage, but to underline the maxim that the output should be properly geared and in tune with the decision process as a whole.

THE HALLMARKS OF RATIONALITY

It is sensible to analyse the decision process in all its ramifications only against the assumption of rational behaviour on the part of the decision-maker. If he behaves irrationally, namely if he does not (when he makes a resolution) abide by an agreed criterion that specifies how a choice between alternatives is to be made, then much of what is accomplished in the preceding stages of the decision process may be irrelevant or immaterial to his final resolution. Consequently, rationality in this context is best defined by reference to the decision process itself: each time the final resolution deviates from what would be expected from following the process, then the resolution cannot be said to be rational.

The decision-maker may argue that though his resolution does not conform to the official decision process, it should still be regarded as rational, because it would conform if an alternative decision process is agreed upon, namely a procedure that he approves of. But the question still remains: Does he or does he not adhere to this alternative decision process? If he does, namely if it is possible to discern such an alternative process (which we may conveniently term "the informal decision process," as opposed to the formal, or official, one) then the decision-maker acts rationally from his viewpoint, but alas irrationally from the organisation's viewpoint. If, on the other hand, this alternative decision process has not been clearly prespecified and is little more than a figment of the decision-maker's imagination, then his behaviour is irrational from every viewpoint.

Determination of Choice Criteria

A distinction must, therefore, be made between the situation where the decision-maker has been responsible for or a party to the determination of the choice criterion and the situation where he has not. In the latter, "rationality" and "irrationality" must be judged with reference either to the organisation or to the individual decision-maker. If he makes a resolution that conforms to the criterion imposed by the organisation, but one that he profoundly disagrees with, then from the organisation's viewpoint the resolution is perfectly rational, while from the individual's standpoint it is irrational. If he makes a resolution that conforms to his own criterion in opposition to the one specified by the organisation, then the position is reversed. In either case, there is a conflict between the decision-maker and the organisation.

If the decision-maker is responsible for the criterion of choice, the decision process is *personalistic* in character, namely the resolution at the end of the process becomes a function of the decision-maker's own personality, his beliefs, his attitudes and his value judgements. His resolution for given circumstances may well be different from that of another individual, though both may still behave rationally by our definition. If, on the other hand, the decision-maker does not participate in the determination of a choice criterion, the decision process is *impersonalistic* and the outcome must be the same for different decision-makers, if they all behave rationally.

Some Corrolaries of Rational Choice

If the discussion is confined to rational choice, the following observations can be made about the final resolution by the decision-maker:

1. If the decision process produces only one alternative, there can obviously be no free choice exercised by the decision-maker, and therefore no decision. The essence of a *decision* is that the decision-maker has several alternatives open to him, so that he can exercise the prerogative of a conscious choice. In the case of a single alternative being presented, the decision-maker can clearly be dispensed with.

2. If there are several alternatives and if an agreed criterion allows complete ranking in terms of a composite measure of performance (which incorporates several measures or yardsticks), then the ranking process automatically causes one alternative to be superior to others. If the decision-maker behaves rationally, he must resolve to select this superior alternative. In that sense, therefore, he does not really exercise any free choice; the choice has already been made for him by the ranking criterion. Thus, once a choice criterion is agreed upon, the final resolution, or choice, is *automatic*, and again the decision-maker becomes redundant at that stage of the decision process.

3. If ranking of alternatives is possible and if several alternatives have equal ranking, then the selection criterion fails to discriminate between them. Unless the existing criterion for choice is modified, or a new one is employed, there is no way in which the decision-maker can be guided in giving preference to one alternative over another, and any choice he makes under such conditions may be regarded as a random choice. Once

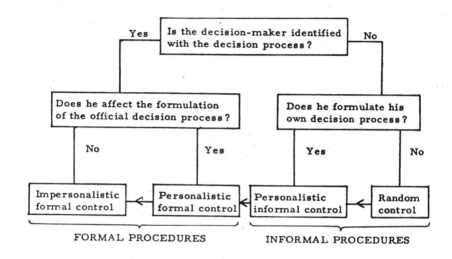

FIGURE 4. Formal and informal procedures

again, the decision-maker is made redundant, since random choices can be made equally well through the use of electro-mechanical devices.

4. If the available information is inadequate, or the analysis of the information is not penetrating enough, to allow the alternative strategies to be ranked at all, then any choice between them can only be made at random, irrespective of how refined and robust the criterion of choice is, and this random choice can be made mechanically.

The perhaps obvious conclusion to be drawn from this discussion is that if a free choice by the decision-maker exists at all, it does not lie at the stage called "resolution" in the decision process, but at the stage where the criterion of choice is determined. If alternatives can be ranked, then for any criterion of choice, resolution is automatic and trivial. The only excuse for including it in the decision process in Figure 1 is to provide a landmark to indicate that the process has come to a final conclusion.

Formal and Informal Procedures

The crux of the decision process lies in the model building stage and in the determination of the criterion of choice. It is mainly in the context of these two stages in the process that the degree of initiative allowed to the decision-maker should be viewed, since these are the significant components in the processes that characterize the control mechanism as being formal or informal, personalistic or impersonalistic (see Figure 4).

The distinction between personalistic and impersonalistic control is somewhat more complicated than suggested in this diagram and a more detailed discussion of this problem is given later, but crude as it is the diagram suggests an interesting hierarchy of four control procedures. Random control is at one extreme end of the scale and impersonalistic-formal control at the other. Observations of the development of control procedures in industry suggest that they have a tendency to move in a direction shown by the arrows: Starting with a situation in which decisions and corrective actions are taken in a haphazard fashion (random control) in the absence of any directives, an individual emerges and tried to regularise these actions and mould them into a systematic and consistent pattern. As long as his procedure does not have the formal blessing of the organisation, it may be characterised as personalistic-informal. Subsequently the procedure is formalised and when eventually it tends to be independent of the individual it becomes impersonalistic-formal. The growth of enterprises from family concerns to large companies, the introduction of computer systems, the aftermath of developing a new product—all these are examples in which process of formalisation and impersonalisation can very often be detected.

Maximising Utility

So far the discussion of rationality has been confined to the final stages of the decision process. But what about the earlier stages? One way of considering a decision-maker who is engaged in constructing a model and weighing alternative strategies, is to regard him as a problem solver. When is his behaviour as a problem solver to be regarded as rational? Von Neumann and Morgenstern briefly discuss the concept of rationality in problem solving and say that an individual who attempts to obtain the maximum utility is said to act rationally and this definition is not at variance with the one suggested here. They go on to say:

> But it may safely be stated that there exists, at present, no satisfactory treatment of the question of rational behavior. There may, for example, exist several ways by which to reach the optimum position; they may depend on the knowledge and understanding which the individual has and upon the paths of action open to him. [6, p. 9]

There may be an implication in this statement that rationality is to be regarded as a function of the method used to arrive at the optimum solution, that if an optimum solution to a problem exists, an individual is said to behave rationally if he arrives at the solution through the use of the best (most efficient?) generally known method. This train of thought would suggest that rationality should be defined in absolute terms, which are determined by the problem and by the general consensus of opinion as to how to solve it, so that if an individual is seen to follow this path, his behaviour is considered to be rational.

This is certainly not the implication that I wish to convey in the definition of rationality suggested here. If an individual fails to follow the generally accepted path because of his ignorance of the existence of this path, and if he persists in following his own path, then from his point of view he behaves perfectly rationally, even if he does not attain the best solution and even if his actions appear to make no sense to a knowledgeable outsider. It seems to me that the first statement of von Neumann and Morgenstern is adequate to describe rationality in the context of this discussion, namely that *an individual is said to behave rationally if he attempts to obtain the maximum utility*. Rationality is, therefore, a relative concept. What is utility to one individual (let alone maximum utility) may not be utility to another. In a personalistic type of control the goals, the utilities, the criterion of choice between alternatives and the final result of the decision process, may be very different for different individuals, even though all may behave rationally in the context of the definition given here.

The Method of Solution

What happens, one might ask, when an individual has followed his own method of solution and refuses to adopt what is generally acknowledged to be a superior method, in other words the individual can no longer argue that he is unaware of the existence of this other method? Does he behave rationally?

The answer, it seems to me, lies in whether the alleged superior method yields a better solution or not. The criterion as to what is "better" has already been determined and agreed by the individual prior to or in the course of his following his own path to arrive at a solution. If a new method is brought to his attention and is shown to produce a better result, better as judged by this criterion, and if the individual persists in ignoring this method, how can he claim to act rationally? In our definition, he no longer attempts to obtain the maximum utility, and therefore he ceases to behave rationally.

If, on the other hand, the new method produces the same or as good a solution as the one derived by the individual's method, then superiority of one method over another can be claimed only on grounds of efficiency (speed of calculations or economy in procedure), rigour, convenience or elegance. And here the answer to the question whether the individual continues to behave rationally depends on whether he accepts these arguments. If he does, yet refuses to change his method, he is irrational; if he does not, his behaviour from his viewpoint continues to be rational, though to others it may seem rather eccentric.

FREEDOM OF CHOICE

The many references to the ability of an individual to make a choice from among a number of available alternatives naturally raises the question: How and under what circumstances can an individual be said to have a freedom of choice?

This problem has exercised the minds of philosophers throughout the ages and has been the subject of numerous treatises. Of all the various approaches to this subject I have chosen to discuss here briefly the view of Ofstad, who provides a comprehensive review of the literature on this topic and suggests his own definition of freedom of choice.

Ofstad's View

Ofstad discusses freedom from determinism (or "freedom as indeterminancy", as he puts it) at some length [4, chapter III] and proceeds to consider four other possible definitions of free will: "freedom as self-expression," "freedom as rationality," "freedom as virtue" and "freedom as power." Some of the arguments under these various headings are very closely related to the discussion on determinism, others are covered in my previous discussion of the concepts of rationality and personalistic control and need not concern us any further here. What is, perhaps, more interesting is that after a detailed discourse of free will in relation to ethical criteria, Ofstad concludes with his own definition of a free person:

> P is a *free person* if, and only if, the following three conditions are fulfilled: (1) P's ethical system is oriented towards such values as love, tolerance and human dignity, (2) he has knowledge of his ethical system, his motivation and choice-situations so that he is able to find out which course of action will be best in accordance with this system, and (3) he is so strongly and whole-heartedly disposed to decide in favor of the course of action which he believes to be the right one, that he does not have to make any efforts in order to decide. [4, pp. 305–306]

This definition is not very satisfactory. The first condition requires definition of love, tolerance and human dignity, and above all it requires a definition of the degrees of orientation towards these values that would allow a person to be identified as free or otherwise. The second condition imposes similar difficulties of definition: what level of intimate knowledge does a person have to possess of his ethical system, motivation and alternative strategies to satisfy this condition? And do we ever get a situation where full knowledge of these issues does in fact exist? The first part of condition (3) is reminiscent of what I called personalistic control, but the second part is too ambiguous to be helpful: if the individual does not require to make any effort to make a decision, then the implication is that the outcomes of possible alternatives have already been arranged in a complete ranking order and in terms of Fig. 1 all that is left is to make the final selection, which then—as already pointed out—becomes a trivial component in the decision process.

One implication of Ofstad's definition is that freedom of choice is a matter of degree, and while we have as yet no way of ranking this degree of freedom (except, perhaps, in some trivial cases), the notion of partial freedom may be thought by some to be useful. As Ofstad says in his preface:

> Power to decide is not something which we have either in full or not at all. It is a matter of degrees and individual variations. What one man can do is not necessarily what another can do. What we can do in one situation may be different from what we can accomplish in another. [4, p. ix]

The other implication of Ofstad's definition, in the context of our discussion of the decision process, is that personalistic control does (or may) involve free choice whereas impersonalistic control does not (this is my own interpretation) and this is an implication that I fully endorse. It seems, however, that this result may be obtained by adopting the definition that freedom of choice exists when an individual has two or more alternative courses of action available to him and when there is no external compulsion to choose a particular alternative. This definition avoids many of the difficulties that are presented by a wider concept based on the absence of compulsion (some of these difficulties were discussed earlier) and it ignores the circumstances that have led to delimiting the range of available alternatives. Admittedly, if two individuals P_1 and P_2 are placed in identical situations and if P_1 is allowed three alternative courses of action and P_2 is allowed only two, then P_1's scope is wider than that of P_2. However, *both individuals are free to make a choice*. Some concept to indicate and even to measure this difference in scope would, therefore, be useful and while I am not proposing to define such a concept here, I suggest that it need not be part of the definition of freedom of choice.

ON UTILITY

The criterion of choice involves the determination of a measure of utility which incorporates the various entities defined as measures of performance and gives expression to the objective that the decision process is designed to attain. Take, for example, a production system in which capacity constraints lead to a conflict between several products. If the measures of performance are defined as the profit values for these products, and if the profit for one product can be increased at the expense of that derived from another product, then the purpose of the single utility scale is to take account of all the individual measures of performance, and in the example cited it may simply be the algebraic sum of all the profit values. If the total profit for all the products is defined as the utility function, and thereby implies that the objective of the decision process is to secure as high a value of this function as possible, then the decision-maker need no longer consider the effect of possible strategies on any one particular product; the conflict between the products is reconciled by the introduction of the utility scale.

Or take the case of controlling inventory to meet variable demand. If stock is depleted, demand cannot be met and if customers are not prepared to wait until the stock is replenished, then loss of revenue is incurred during the stock runout period, coupled with a loss in customer goodwill. The incidence of runouts (or alternatively, the percentage of the amount of stock not available on demand) can be reduced if the average stock holding is increased. The relationship between these two performance measures is shown in Figure 5, where strategy 1 associated with R_1 of runouts requires Q_1 average stock level and is compared with strategy 2, for which the corresponding values are R_2 and Q_2 respectively and $R_1 > R_2$ but $Q_2 > Q_1$. If both measures can be translated to cost figures, for example by considering linear cost parameters a and b for the two measures respectively (namely a is the cost of increasing runout incidence by one unit and b is the cost of increasing the average stock level by one unit), then the utility function becomes $aR_1 + bQ_1$ for strategy 1 and $aR_2 + bQ_2$ for strategy 2 and the one that has the lower value (since the implied objective is to minimise the total cost) is preferable.

It may be useful to pause here and state some axioms and corrolaries associated with utility theory and which are due to von Neumann and Morgenstern [6, chapter 3]:

1. If there are two entities u and v and an individual is asked to state his preference, then only one of three relationships exists:

   $u > v$ which means that he prefers u to v
   $u < v$ which means that he prefers v to u
   $u = v$ which means that he has no preference, namely both are equally desirable or undesirable.

2. If there are three entities u, v and w and if he states that $u > w$ and $w > v$, then $u > v$. This axiom implies transitivity of preference.

3. A weighting parameter α is defined in the interval $0 < \alpha < 1$. If there are three entities $u > w > v$ then a number α exists such that

(1) $$\alpha u + (1 - \alpha)v = w$$

i.e. u and v are given complimentary weights, such that the decision-maker becomes indifferent to the weighted sum or to w. Similarly, a value of α exists so that

(2) $$\alpha u + (1 - \alpha)v > w$$

and a value of α also exists so that

(3) $$\alpha u + (1 - \alpha)v < w.$$

It follows that if there are three entities $u = w = v$, then equation (1) is true for any value of α.

4. If there are two entities $u > v$ then

(4) $$v > \alpha u + (1 - \alpha) v > u$$

for any value of α (in the prescribed interval 0 to 1).

5. If there are n entities or utilities u_1, u_2, $\cdots$, u_n such that for any three entities a number α exists to produce a relationship as stated in equation (1), then the n entities can be arranged in a complete ranking order.

It should, perhaps, be pointed out that in discussing the parameter α von Neumann and Morgenstern often refer to it as a measure of probability. Thus, if there are two possible outcomes to a given course of action and the corresponding utilities of these outcomes are u and v respectively then the expression $\alpha u + (1 - \alpha)v$ states the combination of these two events when α and $1 - \alpha$ are their respective probabilities. This combination describes the *expected utility* of the two possible events and, as we shall see later, allows for alternative strategies to be compared when each strategy may result in one of several outcomes and when each outcome has a single utility. By not specifically stating that α is a measure of probability, it is possible to extend these considerations to the case where each outcome or event has several utilities associated with it.

Let us now examine the way in which such a theory of utility can be applied for single and multiple objectives in deterministic and probabilistic systems.

1. *Deterministic outcomes with a single objective.* Suppose that a decision-maker has m strategies to choose from and a single measure of

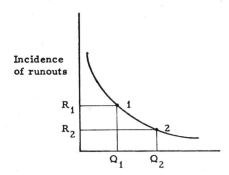

Incidence
of runouts

R_1 —— 1

R_2 —— 2

Q_1 Q_2

FIGURE 5. Trading-off stock level
against stock runout

performance has been defined. If we consider for a moment a deterministic system, so that the utility (described by the measure of performance) or the outcome for each strategy is known, then the decision-maker's task is reduced to identifying the highest utility from an array of m values (each corresponding to one of the strategies), and as the theory of utility assumes that complete ranking is possible, there is no difficulty for the decision-maker in completing his task.

2. *Deterministic outcomes with multiple objective.* What we often encounter in reality is the existence of multiple objectives, as we have seen from the few examples cited earlier. Let us confine our discussion to the deterministic case and consider a set of N measures of performance that are assigned to each course of action. For any given strategy there are N utilities $u_1, u_2, \cdots, u_N$ that describe the corresponding outcome.

The result of arranging N utilities $u_1, u_2, \cdots, u_N$ in a complete ranking order and the computation of weighting parameters, such as α in equation (1), is to produce a set of weighting constants $a_1, a_2, \cdots, a_N$ so that the composite utility U becomes the weighted sum of the N utilities

$$(5) \qquad U = a_1 u_1 + a_2 u_2 + \cdots + a_N u_N.$$

If this utility function U is computed for all the available alternative strategies, the results for U can be arranged in a complete ranking order and the best strategy is then immediately identified. This is shown in Table 1 which consists of m rows for m alternative strategies; each row lists N utilities for any one strategy, so that U_{ij} is the utility j for performance measure j, and the composite utility U_i for strategy i is given in the last column. The values of U_i are all related to one composite numerical scale and the one with the highest value signifies the best strategy that should be selected.

3. *Probabilistic outcomes with a single objective.* The discussion so

TABLE 1
A Utility Table

Measures of Performance........	1	2	...	j	N	Composite Utility
Weights.....	a_1	a_2	...	a_j	a_N	
Strategies 1	u_{11}	u_{12}		u_{1j}	u_{1N}	U_1
$\vdots$ i $\vdots$	...			u_{ij}		U_i
m	...				u_{mN}	U_m

far has been confined to decision making under conditions of certainty, namely each strategy is assumed to be associated with a particular outcome. If only a single measure of performance applies, then ordering the strategies on a scale is automatic; if several measures of performance have to be considered, the reconciliation between them follows equation (5) and Table 1.

What happens under conditions of risk, when the outcome of any particular strategy is associated with a known probability? It is not difficult to see that composite utilities can be constructed in a similar way. Take first the case of a single measure of performance, so that u_j is the utility of outcome j. In Table 2 there are m strategies and n outcomes and the probability matrix p_{ij} is the probability that strategy i will lead to outcome j.

The expected utility from strategy 1 is

$$(6) \qquad U_1 = p_{11}u_1 + p_{12}u_2 + \cdots + p_{1j}u_j + \cdots + p_{1n}u_n$$

where

$$p_{11} + p_{12} + \cdots + p_{ij} + \cdots + p_{1n} = 1$$

and similarly the expected utility for each of the m strategies can be found. There is a certain analogy between Table 1 and Table 2 and between equations (5) and (6). In view of the axioms enumerated earlier, the values of U_i can be ordered on a ranking scale and the optimal strategy can therefore be immediately identified.

4. *Probabilistic outcomes with multiple objectives.* The case of multi-performance measures is handled in the following way: A utility matrix is constructed similar to Table 1. Composite utilities are then calculated for the various outcomes and these are fed as the utility values in Table 2, from which the expected utilities for the available strategies are computed. The procedure is summarised in Table 3, in which, for conveni-

TABLE 2

Probability Matrix for a Single Measure of Performance

Outcomes		1	2	$\cdots$	j	$\cdots$	n	Total Prob.	Expected Utility
Utility		u_1	u_2	$\cdots$	u_j	$\cdots$	u_n		
Strategies	1	p_{11}	p_{12}		p_{1j}		p_{1n}	1	U_1
	$\vdots$								
	i	$\cdots$			p_{ij}		$\cdots$	1	U_i
	$\vdots$								
	m	$\cdots$					p_{mn}	1	U_m

ence of presentation, the top part is an inverted version of Table 1 (i.e. now each column enumerates the utilities for the corresponding outcome) and the bottom part duplicates Table 2.

The Notion of Probability

Circumstances of risk are characterised by the fact that the matrix of decisions and outcomes has occurred many times in the past and that the general pattern of events suggests that steady state conditions prevail to allow an inference for future outcomes to be based on frequencies of past events. But such conditions rarely exist in a business environment, where decisions have to be made under conditions of uncertainty rather than risk, namely where probabilities of future outcomes cannot be equated to frequencies of past outcomes, either because such information is too meagre or nonexistent, or because present and future circumstances are believed to be significantly different from the past.

Diverse and often conflicting views are found among decision theorists on how to handle decision making under conditions of uncertainty. Some suggest methods for determining subjective probability measures, with which the problem of uncertainty can then be handled as if conditions of known risk prevail. Others argue that the conventional concept of probability be abandoned and that other procedures should be employed in order to compare the relative merit of outcomes and hence to identify the most desirable strategy. A fairly detailed account of the various schools of thought on this subject is given by Fishburn [3, Chapter 5] and this is not an appropriate place to elaborate on the subject, except to draw attention to the fact that fundamental differences in points of view are very much in existence.

It should perhaps also be pointed out that the very issue of whether a given situation may be described as one of risk or uncertainty is often also open to judgement and dispute. When it comes to making inferences about

TABLE 3

The Case of Multi-Performance Measures Under Conditions of Risk

Outcomes		1	j	n	Weights
Measures of	1				a_1
performance	$\vdots$				$\vdots$
	k		u_{kj}		a_k
	$\vdots$				$\vdots$
	N				a_N
Outcomes Composite		u_1	u_j	u_n	

$\downarrow$

Outcomes....................	1	j	n	Total	Expected Utility
Composite Utility...............	u_1	u_j	u_n		
Strategies 1				1	U_1
$\vdots$					$\vdots$
i		p_{ij}		1	U_i
$\vdots$					$\vdots$
m				1	U_m

the future, historical records may well be interpreted in several ways, let alone the challenge that may be levelled at the assertion that such inference is at all valid. What seems to one individual a perfectly legitimate case of decision under risk may be argued by another as being a case of uncertainty, and the case of uncertainty is then amenable to interpretation in several ways, depending on the school of thought that the individual professes to be a disciple of.

THE RELATION BETWEEN UTILITY THEORY AND RATIONALITY

To summarize for the purpose of this discussion, the significant assumptions in the theory of utility suggested by von Neumann and Morgenstern are:
   (a) An individual is capable of ranking utilities. This assumption also implies consistency, or the need to avoid contradiction: If he prefers u to v then he cannot at the same time prefer v to u or be indifferent as to which utility he prefers.
   (b) There is transitivity of preference.

(c) Weighting factors can be determined to compare utilities and
    hence to establish a composite utility scale.

It is worthwhile repeating these assumptions because of the significance that has been attributed to these axioms in relation to the concept of
rationality. Von Neumann and Morgenstern lay great emphasis on the
need for quantitative measurements in economics and after discussing
their proposed axioms state that their purpose is "to find the mathemati-
cally complete principles which define 'rational behavior' for the participants in a social economy, and to derive from them the general characteristics of that behavior" [6, p. 31]. Many decision theorists go further and
specifically identify the axioms of utility theory as axioms of rational
behaviour.

By this test most decisions in reality will probably have to be regarded
as irrational. Take, for example, the assumption that by assigning appropriate weights a multiobjective array can be transformed to a single measure on a composite utility scale. Individuals may have very strong views
about the desirability of attaining each of the stated objectives, but may
find it impossible to compare and reconcile them.

When, in As You Like It, Corin asked Touchstone "and how like you
this shepherd's life?", Touchstone replied:

> Truly shepherd, in respect of itself, it is a good life; but in respect that it is
> a shepherd's life, it is naught. In respect that it is solitary, I like it very
> well: but in respect that it is private, it is a very vile life. Now in respect it
> is in the fields, it pleaseth me well: but in respect it is not in the Court, it is
> tedious. As it is a spare life (look you) it fits my humour well: but as there
> is no more plenty in it, it goes much against my stomach. Hast any
> philosophy in thee shepherd? [5]

In terms of any one objective an individual may find it possible to rank
alternatives without much difficulty, but when it comes to declaring how
much he is prepared to trade off one utility against another, he may be
quite helpless.

Or suppose, for the sake of argument, that a man is faced with the
prospect of enjoying the company of one of three ladies, A, B, or C. He can
enumerate many of the qualities of these splendid ladies—their physical
dimensions, the complexion of their skins, the colour of their eyes, their
I.Q.'s, the number of pimples per square inch, etc.—but he finds it impossible to come up with a composite measure of utility. The whole idea of a
trade off between any two qualities he finds totally unacceptable. How is
he to equate the level of intellect with the density of pimples, he asks? The
utility of any one quality may well depend on the presence of other
qualities. For example, he may regard a high density of pimples a positive

asset when accompanied with certain skin and hair colouring, but a liability in other combinations. Nevertheless, he feels that he can compare two ladies at a time on the basis of an overall evaluation. If, having done this, he states that he prefers A to B and B to C and C to A, he does not abide by the axiom of transitivity of preference. The violation of this axiom undermines the elegant mathematical structure of utility theory and many decision theorists have no patience for such an individual and would simply regard him as irrational.

It should perhaps be pointed out that a "circular ranking," such as the one just described, does not necessarily violate the axiom of consistency. Our man may be perfectly consistent in always preferring (within a given space of time) A to B, etc., and avoiding any contradiction between any of two of his statements. Admittedly, faced with a set of preferences as stated so far, he is unable to make a choice, since for any choice that he makes a better one (as judged by his own preferences) can be pointed out. Does the fact that he cannot act prove that he is irrational? In our discussion we have drawn a distinction between the determination of choice criteria and the act of selecting between alternatives; our man can argue that he truly *attempts to obtain the maximum utility* (which is our definition of rational behaviour), but the choice criteria do not provide him with a means of making a final selection.

To base a concept of rationality on the axioms of utility theory that were listed earlier is therefore to take a rather narrow view and to exclude from the realm of rationality a significant proportion of decisions that do take place in daily life.

Let us now return to further considerations of personalistic control.

PERSONALISTIC AND IMPERSONALISTIC CONTROL

A distinction was made in Figure 4 between personalistic and impersonalistic control by examining whether an individual does or does not affect the formulation of the decision process. In the light of the foregoing discussion it would appear that personalistic and impersonalistic control are not two entirely mutually exclusive categories, but that several shades and degrees of personalistic involvement in the decision process can be identified. Consider the following two groups of questions about an individual:

Group (a): First order of personalistic involvement:

1. Does the individual set up the number and identity of the measures of performance?

2. In case of multi-objectives, does he specify the weighting coefficients that determine the composite utility function? If this is not possible, does he rank the outcomes and does he determine the criterion of choice?
3. Does he specify the array of available strategies?
4. Does he specify the array of possible outcomes?
5. Does he specify whether the decision making process does or does not take place under conditions of certainty?

Group (b): Second order of personalistic involvement (when the decision is not under conditions of certainty):

6. Does he specify which decision theory to apply?
7. If probabilities of possible outcomes are required for the decision process, does he determine their values?
8. Does he determine the value of any subjective parameters (other than probabilities) that may be required in the application of a given decision theory (e.g. the coefficient of optimism if the Hurwicz criterion is adopted)?

Group (a) consists of questions that may be posed for every decision process. Group (b) is only relevant if the decision process is not subject to conditions of certainty.

There are four possible answers to each of these eight questions:

Yes—   where the individual does carry out the activity described in the question, and even if his specification may subsequently be modified in the light of criticisms and suggestions by other people, these modifications are comparatively slight or the responsibility for the final specifications clearly lies with the individual.

No—   when the specifications described by the question are laid down or are the responsibility of someone else, or when they are covered by standing orders and procedures.

Participates—   when the individual is a member of a group of people responsible for the activity described in the question (e.g. when the group is a committee, or when specifications are based on averages of values suggested by several individuals).

Irrelevant—   when the question does not apply (any one or several of questions 2, 6, 7 and 8 may become irrelevant in the light of answers to the other questions).

It should be emphasised that answers to the eight questions are to some extent a matter of subjective interpretation on the part of the questioner or investigator. It may be difficult in some circumstances to determine whether an individual should give the first or the third answer to a particular question. Nevertheless, the purpose of these questions is not to compute a crisp numerical value for the level of personalistic involvement of a particular individual, but to produce a profile of his involvement, as demonstrated by the answers in the example shown below (pertaining to a given task or decision process):

Question	Answer		
1	N		
2	P		
3	Y	Legend:	Y—yes
4	Y		N—no
5	N		P—participates
6	N		— —question irrelevant
7	P		
8	—		

If answers to relevant questions are all "no," then control is strictly formal and impersonalistic, if all the answers are "yes" then control is purely personalistic, and between these two extremes there is a whole spectrum of alternative combinations.

It is in this context that the tendency of a decision process to become formal and impersonalistic in character may be traced: if answers to the eight questions are monitored over a period of time, then this tendency can be documented, as in the example below:

Question	Time→			
1	N	N	N	N
2	P	N	N	N
3	Y	Y	N	N
4	Y	Y	Y	P
5	N	N	N	N
6	N	N	N	N
7	P	P	N	N
8	—	—	—	—

Where Does the Decision Lie?

Having examined the various stages of the decision process, we may now return to Figure 1 and ask: Where are the crucial points in this process? Where can the decision maker be said to affect the turn of events?

The answer lies in the degree of personalistic control that he retains. We have already seen how a data processing facility can encroach on the decision-maker's domain by taking over parts or the whole function of analysis. Similarly, when the decision process as a whole becomes more and more impersonalistic, it simply follows the rules, and the rules are sufficiently detailed to cater for an ever increasing number of contingencies to obliterate the effect of the individual decision-maker. In the extreme case, when control is completely impersonalistic, the decision-maker ceases to have a meaningful role; he ceases to be a decision-maker.

References

1. Churchman, C. W., *Challenge to reason*, McGraw Hill, 1968.
2. Eilon, S., "Some notes on information processing," *Journal of Management Studies*, Vol. 5, No. 2 (1968), pp. 139–153.
3. Fishburn, P.C., *Decision and value theory*, Wiley, 1964.
4. Ofstad, H., *An inquiry into the freedom of decision*, Allen and Unwin, 1961.
5. Shakespeare, W., *As you like it*, Act 3, Scene 3, 1623.
6. Von Neumann, J. and Morgenstern, O., *Theory of games and economic behavior*, Princeton Univ. Press, 1953.

16

On the Concept of
Organizational Goal

HERBERT A. SIMON

Few discussions of organization theory manage to get along without introducing some concept of "organization goal." In the classical economic
theory of the firm, where no distinction is made between an organization
and a single entrepreneur, the organization's goal—the goal of the firm—is
simply identical with the goal of the real or hypothetical entrepreneur. In
general, it is thought not to be problematical to postulate that individuals
have goals. If it is not, this solution raises no difficulties.

When we are interested in the internal structure of an organization,
however, the problem cannot be avoided in this way. Either we must
explain organizational behavior in terms of the goals of the individual
members of the organization, or we must postulate the existence of one or
more organization goals, over and above the goals of the individuals.[1]

The first alternative is an attractive one. It protects us from the
danger of reifying the organization, of treating it as a superindividual

---

[1] The present discussion is generally compatible with, but not identical to, that of my
colleagues, R. M. Cyert and J. G. March, who discuss organizational goals in ch. iii of *A
Behavioral Theory of the Firm* (Englewood Cliffs, N.J., 1963). Their analysis is most
germane to the paragraphs of this paper that treat of motivation for goals and organizational
survival.

FROM: *Administrative Science Quarterly*, Vol. 4, June 1964, pp. 1-22.

entity having an existence and behavior independent of the behavior of its members. The difficulty with this alternative is that it is hard to carry off. The usual way it is attempted is by identifying the phrase "organization goals" with "goals of the firm's owners" or, alternatively, "goals of the firm's top management," or "goals of those who hold legitimate authority to direct the organization."

But this solution raises new difficulties, for we often have occasion to observe that the goals that actually underlie the decisions made in an organization do not coincide with the goals of the owners, or of top management, but have been modified by managers and employees at all echelons. Must we conclude, then, that it is the goals of the latter—of subordinate managers and employees—that are governing organizational behavior? Presumably not, because the kinds of behavior taking place are not those we would expect if the managers and employees were consulting only their personal goals. The whole concept of an informal organization, modified by, but not identical with, the goals either of management or of individual employees, becomes hazy and ambiguous if we follow this path.

Let us see if we can find a way between this Scylla and the Charybdis of reification. The first step toward clarification is to maintain a distinction between goals, on the one hand, and motives, on the other. By *goals* we shall mean value premises that can serve as inputs to decisions. By *motives* we mean the causes, whatever they are, that lead individuals to select some goals rather than others as premises for their decisions. In the next section we shall develop the concept of goal, defined as above. In subsequent sections we shall undertake to explicate the notion of *organization goal* and to clarify the relations between organization goals and personal motives.

Before we can define "organization goals" we shall have to be clear on what we mean by "goals of an individual." We shall begin by considering the latter question.

GOALS AND DECISIONS: MULTIPLE CRITERIA

Our discussion of goals will be much simplified if we have a definite model before us of the situation we are considering. In recent years in the field of management science or operations research, we have learned to build formal models to characterize even quite elaborate and complex decision situations, and to use these models to reach "optimal" decisions. Since many of these models make use of the tool of linear programming, we will employ a linear programming framework to describe the decision situation. No mathematical knowledge will be assumed beyond the ability to read algebraic notation.[2]

The optimal diet problem is a typical simple linear programming problem. We are given a list of foods, and for each item on the list its price, its calory content, and its proportions of each of the minerals and vitamins relevant to nutrition. Then we are given a set of nutritional requirements, which may include statements about minimum daily intake of minerals, vitamins, and calories, and may also put limits on maximum intake of some or all of these components.

The diet problem is to find that sublist of foods and their quantities that will meet the nutritional requirements at least cost. The problem can be formalized as follows:

Let the various foods be numbered from 1 through N, and the various nutritional components from 1 through M. Let x_i be the quantity of the ith food in the diet, y_j be the total quantity of the jth nutritional component in the diet, and p_i the price of the ith food. Let a_{ij} be the amount of the jth nutritional component in a unit quantity of the ith food; let b_j be the minimum requirement of the jth nutritional component, and c_j the maximum allownace. (Some of the b_j's may be zero, and some of the c_j's infinite.) Then:

(1) $$\sum_i a_{ij} x_i = y_j, \quad \text{for } j = 1, \ldots, M;$$

i.e., the total consumption of the jth nutritional element is the sum of the quantities of that element for each of the foods consumed. The nutritional requirements can be stated:

(2) $$c_j \geq y_j \geq b_j, \quad \text{for } j = 1, \ldots, M;$$

i.e., the total quantity of the jth element must lie between b_j and c_j. The quantity of each food consumed must be non-negative, although it may be zero:

(3) $$x_i \geq 0, \quad i = 1, \ldots, N.$$

---

[2] There are now a substantial number of elementary discussions of linear programming in the management science literature. For a treatment that develops the point of view proposed here, see A. Charnes and W. W. Cooper, *Management Models and Industrial Applications of Linear Programming* (New York, 1961), ch. i. See also Charnes and Cooper, Deterministic Equivalents for Optimizing and Satisfying under Chance Constraints, *Operations Research*, 11 (1963), 18–39.

Finally, the total cost of the diet is to be minimized; we are to find:

(4) $$\text{Min}_x \sum_i x_i p_i.$$

A diet (the solution is not necessarily unique) that satisfies all the relations (2), (3), (4) is called an *optimal* diet. A diet that satisfies the inequalities (2) and (3) (called *constraints*), but which is not necessarily a minimum cost diet, is called a *feasible* diet.

What is the goal of the diet decision? It would be an appropriate use of ordinary language to say that the goal is to minimize the cost of obtaining an adequate diet, for the condition (4) is the criterion we are minimizing. This criterion puts the emphasis on economy as the goal.

Alternatively, we might direct our attention primarily to the constraints, and in particular to the nutritional requirements (2). Then we might say that the goal is to find a nutritionally satisfactory diet that is economical. Although we still mention costs in this statement, we have clearly shifted the emphasis to the adequacy of the diet from a nutritional standpoint. The primary goal has now become good nutrition.

The relation between the criterion function (4) and the constraints (2) can be made even more symmetrical. Let us replace the criterion (4) with a new constraint:

(5) $$\sum_i x_i p_i \leqq k,$$

that is to say, with the requirement that the total cost of the diet not exceed some constant, k. Now the set of feasible diets has been restricted to those that satisfy (5) as well as (2) and (3). But since the minimization condition has been removed, there is apparently no basis for choosing one of these diets over another.

Under some circumstances, we can, however, restrict the set of diets that deserve consideration to a subset of the feasible set. Suppose that all the nutritional constraints (2) are minimal constraints, and that we would always prefer, *ceteris paribus*, a greater amount of any nutritional factor to a smaller amount. We will say that diet A is dominated by diet B if the cost of diet B is no greater than the cost of diet A, and if diet B contains at least as much of each nutritional factor as does diet A, and more of at least one factor. We will call the set of diets in the feasible set that is undominated by other diets in that set the Pareto optimal set.

Our preference for one or the other of the diets in the Pareto optimal set will depend on the relative importance we assign to cost in comparison with amounts of nutritional factors, and to the amounts of these factors in relation with each other. If cost is the most important factor, then we will again choose the diet that is selected by criterion (4). On the other hand, if we attach great importance to nutritional factor j, we will generally choose a quite different feasible diet—one in which the quantity of factor j is as great as possible. Within the limits set by the constraints, it would be quite reasonable to call whatever criterion led us to select a particular member of the Pareto optimal set our goal. But if the constraints are strong enough, so that the feasible set and, *a fortiori*, the Pareto optimal is set very small, then the constraints will have as much or more influence on what diet we finally select than will the goal, so defined. For example, if we set one or more of the nutritional requirements very high, so that only a narrow range of diets also satisfy the budget constraint (5), then introducing the cost minimization criterion as the final selection rule will have relatively little effect on what diet we choose.

Under such circumstances it might be well to give up the idea that the decision situation can be described in terms of a simple goal. Instead, it would be more reasonable to speak of a whole set of goals—the whole set, in fact, of nutritional and budgetary constraints—that the decision maker is trying to attain. To paraphrase a familiar epigram: "If you allow me to determine the constraints, I don't care who selects the optimization criterion."

MULTIPLE CRITERIA IN ORGANIZATIONS

To show the organizational relevance of our example it is only necessary to suppose that the decision we are discussing has arisen within a business firm that manufactures commercial stock feeds, that the nutritional requirements are requirements for hogs and the prices those of available feed ingredients, and that the finished feed prices facing the firm are fixed. Then minimizing the cost of feed meeting certain nutritional standards is identical with maximizing the profit from selling feed meeting those standards. Cost minimization represents the profit-maximizing goal of the company.

We can equally well say that the goal of the feed company is to provide its customers with the best feed possible, in terms of nutritional standards, at a given price, i.e., to produce feeds that are in the Pareto optimal set. Presumably this is what industry spokesmen mean when they say that the goal of business is not profit but efficient production of goods and services. If we had enlarged our model to give some of the prices that appear in it the status of constraints, instead of fixing them as constants, we could have introduced other goals, for example, the goal of suppliers' profits, or, if there were a labor input, the goal of high wages.[3]

---

[3] See "A Comparison of Organization Theories," in my *Models of Man* (New York, 1957), pp. 170–182.

We may summarize the discussion to this point as follows. In the decision-making situations of real life, a course of action, to be acceptable, must satisfy a whole set of requirements, or constraints. Sometimes one of these requirements is singled out and referred to as the goal of the action. But the choice of one of the constraints, from many, is to a large extent arbitrary. For many purposes it is more meaningful to refer to the whole set of requirements as the (complex) goal of the action. This conclusion applies both to individual and organizational decision making.

SEARCH FOR A COURSE OF ACTION

Thus far, we have assumed that the set of possible actions is known in advance to the decision maker. In many, if not most, real-life situations, possible courses of action must be discovered, designed, or synthesized. In the process of searching for a satisfactory solution, the goals of the action—that is, the constraints that must be satisfied by the solution—may play a guiding role in two ways. First, the goals may be used directly to synthesize proposed solutions (*altenative generation*). Second, the goals may be used to test the satisfactoriness of a proposed solution *(alternative testing).*[4]

We may illustrate these possibilities by considering what goes on in the mind of a chess player when he is trying to choose a move in a game. One requirement of a good move is that it put pressure on the opponent by attacking him in some way or by preparing an attack. This requirement suggests possible moves to an experienced player (alternative generation). For example, if the opponent's king is not well protected, the player will search for moves that attack the king, but after a possible move has been generated in this way (and thus automatically satisfies the requirement that it put pressure on the opponent), it must be tested against other requirements (alternative testing). For example, it will not be satisfactory if it permits a counterattack that is more potent than the attack or that can be carried out more quickly.

The decisions of everyday organizational life are similar to these decisions in chess. A bank officer who is investing trust funds in stocks and bonds may, because of the terms of the trust document, take as his goal increasing the capital value of the fund. This will lead him to consider

---

[4] For further discussion of the role of generators and tests in decision making and problem solving, see A. Newell and H. A. Simon, "The Processes of Creative Thinking," in H. E. Gruber, G. Terrell, and M. Wertheimer, eds., *Contemporary Approaches to Creative Thinking* (New York, 1962), particularly pp. 77–91.

buying common stock in firms in growth industries (alternative generation). But he will check each possible purchase against other requirements: that the firm's financial structure be sound, its past earnings record satisfactory, and so on (alternative testing). All these considerations can be counted among his goals in constructing the portfolio, but some of the goals serve as generators of possible portfolios, others as checks.[5]

The process of designing courses of action provides us, then, with another source of asymmetry between the goals that guide the actual synthesis and the constraints that determine whether possible courses of action are in fact feasible. In general, the search will continue until one decision in the feasible set is found, or, at most, a very few alternatives. Which member of the feasible set is discovered and selected may depend considerably on the search process, that is, on which requirements serve as goals or generators, in the sense just defined, and which as constraints or tests.

In a multiperson situation, one man's goals may be another man's constraints. The feed manufacturer may seek to produce feed as cheaply as possible, searching, for example, for possible new ingredients. The feed, however, has to meet certain nutritional specifications. The hog farmer may seek the best quality of feed, searching, for example, for new manufacturers. The feed, however, cannot cost more than his funds allow; if it is too expensive, he must cut quality or quantity. A sale will be made when a lot of feed is feasible in terms of the requirements of both manufacturer and farmer. Do manufacturer and farmer have the same goals? In one sense, clearly not, for there is a definite conflict of interest between them: the farmer wishes to buy cheap, the manufacturer to sell dear. On the other hand, if a bargain can be struck that meets the requirements of both—if the feasible set that satisfies both sets of constraints is not empty—then there is another sense in which they do have a common goal. In the limiting case of perfect competition, the constraints imposed by the market and the technology actually narrow down the feasible set to a single point, determining uniquely the quantity of goods they will exchange and the price.

The neatness and definiteness of the limiting case of perfect competition should not blind us to the fact that most real-life situations do not fit this case exactly. Typically, the generation of alternatives (e.g., product invention, development, and design) is a laborious, costly process. Typically, also, there is a practically unlimited sea of potential alternatives. A river valley development plan that aims at the generation of electric

---

[5] G. P. E. Clarkson, "A Model of Trust Investment Behavior," in Cyert and March, *op. cit.*

power, subject to appropriate provision for irrigation, flood control, and recreation will generally look quite different from a plan that aims at flood control, subject to appropriate provision for the other goals mentioned. Even though the plans generated in both cases will be examined for their suitability along all the dimensions mentioned, it is almost certain that quite different plans will be devised and proposed for consideration in the two cases, and that the plans finally selected will represent quite distinct points in the feasible set.

In later paragraphs we shall state some reasons for supposing that the total sets of constraints considered by decision makers in different parts of an organization are likely to be quite similar, but that different decision makers are likely to divide the constraints between generators and tests in quite different ways. Under these circumstances, if we use the phrase organization goals broadly to denote the constraint sets, we will conclude that organizations do, indeed, have goals (widely shared constraint sets). If we use the phrase organization goals narrowly to denote the generators, we will conclude that there is little communality of goals among the several parts of large organizations and that subgoal formation and goal conflicts are prominent and significant features of organizational life. The distinction we have made between generators and tests helps resolve this ambiguity, but also underlines the importance of always making explicit which sense of goal is intended.

MOTIVATION FOR GOALS

If by motivation we mean whatever it is that causes someone to follow a particular course of action, then every action is motivated—by definition. But in most human behavior the relation between motives and action is not simple; it is mediated by a whole chain of events and surrounding conditions.

We observe a man scratching his arm. His motive (or goal)? To relieve an itch.

We observe a man reaching into a medicine cabinet. His motive (or goal?) To get a bottle of lotion that, his wife has assured him, is very effective in relieving the itch of mosquito bites. Or have we misstated his motive? Is it to apply the lotion to his arm? Or, as before, to relieve the itch? But the connection between action and goal is much more complex in this case than in the previous one. There intervenes between them a means-end chain (get bottle, apply lotion, relieve itch), an expectation (that the lotion will relieve the itch), and a social belief supporting the expectation (that the wife's assurance is a reliable predictor of the lotion's efficacy). The relation between the action and the ultimate goal has become highly indirect and contingent, even in this simple case. Notice that these new complications of indirectness are superimposed on the complications we have discussed earlier—that the goal is pursued only within limits imposed by numerous side constraints (don't knock over the other bottles in the medicine cabinet, don't brush against the fresh paint, and so on).

Our point is identical with the point of the venerable story of the three bricklayers who were asked what they were doing. "Laying bricks," "Building a wall," "Helping to erect a great cathedral," were their respective answers. The investment trust officer whose behavior we considered earlier could answer in any of these modes, or others. "I am trying to select a stock for this investment portfolio." "I am assembling a portfolio that will provide retirement income for my client." "I am employed as an investment trust officer." Now it is the step of indirectness between the second and third answers that has principal interest for organization theory. The investment trust officer presumably has no "personal" interest in the retirement income of his client, only a "professional" interest in his role as trust officer and bank employee. He does have, on the other hand, a personal interest in maintaining that role and that employment status.

ROLE BEHAVIOR

Of course, in real life the line of demarcation between personal and professional interests is not a sharp one, for personal satisfactions may arise from the competent performance of a professional role, and both personal satisfactions and dissatisfactions may result from innumerable conditions that surround the employment. Nevertheless, it is exceedingly important, as a first approximation, to distinguish between the answers to two questions of motive: "Why do you keep (or take) this job?" and "Why do you make this particular investment decision?" The first question is properly answered in terms of the personal motives or goals of the occupant of the role, the second question in terms of goals that define behavior appropriate to the role itself.

Corresponding to this subdivision of goals into personal and role-defined goals, organization theory is sometimes divided into two subparts: (1) a theory of motivation explaining the decisions of people to participate in and remain in organizations; and (2) a theory of decision making within, organizations comprised of such people.[6]

In the motivational theory formulated by Barnard and me, it is post-

---

[6] For further discussion and references, see J. G. March and H. A. Simon, *Organizations* (New York, 1958), ch. iv.

ulated that the motives of each group of participants can be divided into *inducements* (aspects of participation that are desired by the participants) and *contributions* (aspects of participation that are inputs to the organization's production function but that generally have negative utility to participants). Each participant is motivated to maximize, or at least increase, his inducements while decreasing his contributions, and this motivation is a crucial consideration in explaining the decision to join (or remain). But "joining" means accepting an organizational role, and hence we do not need any additional motivational assumptions beyond those of inducements-contributions theory to explain the ensuing role-enacting behavior.

I hasten to repeat the caveat, introduced a few paragraphs above, that in thus separating our consideration of organizational role-enacting behavior from our consideration of personal motivation—allowing the decision to join as the only bridge between them—we are proposing an abstraction from the complexities of real life. A good deal of the significant research on human relations and informal organization, which has contributed heavily in the last generation to our understanding of organizational behavior, has been concerned specifically with the phenomena that this abstraction excludes. Thus, desire for power and concern for personal advancement represent an intrusion of personal goals upon organizational role, as do the social and craft satisfactions and dissatisfactions associated with work.

To say that the abstraction is sometimes untenable is not to deny that there may be many situations in which it is highly useful. There are, first of all, many organizational decisions that simply do not affect personal motives at all—where organizational goals and personal goals are orthogonal, so to speak. As a trivial example, the secretary's inducement-contribution balance is generally in no whit affected by the choice between typing a letter to A or a letter to B or by the content of the letter. Second, personal motives may enter the decision process as fixed constraints (only courses of action that satisfy the constraints are considered, but the constraints have no influence on the choice of action within the set). Thus, the terms of the employment contract may limit work to a forty-hour week but may have little to say about what goes on during the forty hours.[7]

The abstraction of organizational role from personal goals turns out to be particularly useful in studying the cognitive aspects of organizational decision making, for the abstraction is consonant with some known facts about human cognitive processes. Of all the knowledge, attitudes, and values stored in a human memory, only a very small fraction are evoked in

---

[7] See "A Formal Theory of Employment Relation," in *Models of Man*, op. cit.

a given concrete situation. Thus, an individual can assume a wide variety of roles when these are evoked by appropriate circumstances, each of which may interact only weakly with the others. At one time he may be a father, at another a machinist, at another a chess player. Current information processing theories of human cognition postulate that there is only modest overlap of the subsets of memory contents—information and programs—that are evoked by these several roles. Thus, we might postulate that the day-to-day organizational environment evokes quite different associations out of the memory of the participant from those evoked when he is considering a change of jobs. To the extent this is so, it provides a further explanation of why his "personal" system of inducements and contributions, i.e., the utilities that enter into the latter decisions, will have no effect on his "organizational" decisions, i.e., those that are made while the first set is evoked.

The ability of a single individual to shift from one role to another as a function of the environment in which he finds himself thus helps explain the extent to which organizational goals become internalized, that is, are automatically evoked and applied during performance of the role. By whatever means the individual was originally motivated to adopt the role in the first place, the goals and constraints appropriate to the role become a part of the decision-making program, stored in his memory, that defines his role behavior.

INTERPERSONAL DIFFERENCES

Although the considerations introduced in the last section show that the uncoupling of organizational role from personal goals need not be complete, it may be useful to indicate a little more specifically how differences among individuals can affect their behavior in roles that are identical from an organizational standpoint.

A role must be understood not as a specific, stereotyped set of behaviours, but as a *program* (as that word is understood in computer technology) for determining the courses of action to be taken over the range of circumstances that arise. In previous sections we have given examples of such programs and have shown that they can be highly complex; for instance, a single decision may be a function of a large number of program instructions or premises.

Thus, while we may conceive of an ideal type of role that incorporates only organizational goals among its premises, the roles that members of organizations actually enact invariably incorporate both organizational and personal goals. We have already seen how both can be part of the total system of constraints.

But interpersonal differences in the enactment of roles go far beyond the incorporation of personal goals in the role. Role behavior depends on means-end premises as well as goal premises. Thus, particular professional training may provide an individual with specific techniques and knowledge for solving problems (accounting techniques, legal techniques, and so on), which are then drawn upon as part of the program evoked by his role. In this way, a chief executive with an accounting background may find different problem solutions from a chief executive, in the same position, with a legal background.

An individual may incorporate in his role not only a professional style but also a personal style. He may bring to the role, for example, habits and beliefs that provide him with crucial premises for his handling of interpersonal relations. Thus, an authoritarian personality will behave quite differently from a more permissive person when both are in the same organizational role and pursuing the same organizational goals.

The leeway for the expression of individual differences in role behavior is commonly narrowest in the handling of those matters that come to the role occupant at the initiative of others and is commonly broadest in his exercise of initiative and in selecting those discretionary matters to which he will attend and give priority. In terms used in earlier paragraphs, premises supplied by the organizational environment generally control alternative selection more closely than alternative generation.

THE ORGANIZATIONAL DECISION-MAKING SYSTEM

Let us limit ourselves for the present to situations where occupational roles are almost completely divorced from personal goals and pursue the implications of this factoring of the behavior of organizational participants into its personal and organizational components. If we now consider the organizational decision-making programs of all the participants, together with the connecting flow of communication, we can assemble them into a composite description of the organizational decision-making system—a system that has been largely abstracted from the individual motives that determine participation.

In the simplest case, of a small, relatively unspecialized organization, we are back to a decision-making situation not unlike that of the optimal diet problem. The language of "goals," "requirements," "constraints," that we applied there is equally applicable to similarly uncomplicated organizational situations.

In more complicated cases, abstracting out the organizational decision-making system from personal motives does not remove all aspects of interpersonal (more accurately, interrole) difference from the decision-making process. For when many persons in specialized roles participate in making an organization's decisions, the total system is not likely to be monolithic in structure. Individual roles will differ with respect to the number and kinds of communications they receive and the parts of the environment from which they receive them. They will differ with respect to the evaluative communications they receive from other roles. They will differ in their search programs. Hence, even within our abstraction, which neglects personal motives, we can accommodate the phenomena of differential perception and subgoal formation.

To make our discussion more specific, let us again consider a specific example of an organizational decision-making system—in this case a system for controlling inventory and production. We suppose a factory in which decisions have to be made about (1) the aggregate rate of production, that is, the work force that will be employed and the hours employees will work each week, (2) the allocation of aggregate production facilities among the several products the factory makes, and (3) the scheduling of the sequence in which the individual products will be handled on the production facilities. Let us call these the aggregate production decision, item allocation decision, and scheduling decision, respectively. The three sets of decisions may be made by different roles in the organization; in general, we would expect the aggregate decision to be handled at more central levels than the others. The real world situation will always include complications beyond those we have described, for it will involve decisions with respect to shipments to warehouses, decisions as to which products to hold in warehouse inventories, and many others.

Now we could conceive of an omniscient Planner (the entrepreneur of classical economic theory) who, by solving a set of simultaneous equations, would make each and all of these interrelated decisions. Decision problems of this kind have been widely studied during the past decade by management scientists, with the result that we know a great deal about the mathematical structures of the problems and the magnitude of the computations that would be required to solve them. We know, in particular, that discovery of the optimal solution of a complete problem of this kind is well beyond the powers of existing or prospective computational equipment.

In actual organizational practice, no one attempts to find an optimal solution for the whole problem. Instead, various particular decisions, or groups of decisions, within the whole complex are made by specialized members or units of the organization. In making these particular decisions, the specialized units do not solve the whole problem, but find a "satisfactory" solution for one or more subproblems, where some of the effects of the solution on other parts of the system are incorporated in the definition of "satisfactory."

For example, standard costs may be set as constraints for a manufacturing executive. If he finds that his operations are not meeting those constraints, he will search for ways of lowering his costs. Longer production runs may occur to him as a means for accomplishing this end. He can achieve longer production runs if the number of style variations in product is reduced, so he proposes product standardization as a solution to his cost problem. Presumably he will not implement the solution until he has tested it against constraints introduced by the sales department—objections that refusal to meet special requirements of customers will lose sales.

Anyone familiar with organizational life can multiply examples of this sort, where different problems will come to attention in different parts of the organization, or where different solutions will be generated for a problem, depending on where it arises in the organization. The important point to be noted here is that we do not have to postulate conflict in personal goals or motivations in order to explain such conflicts or discrepancies. They could, and would, equally well arise if each of the organizational decision-making roles were being enacted by digital computers, where the usual sorts of personal limits on acceptance of organizational roles would be entirely absent. The discrepancies arise out of the cognitive inability of the decision makers to deal with the entire problem as a set of simultaneous relations, each to be treated symmetrically with the others.[8]

An aspect of the division of decision-making labor that is common to virtually all organizations is the distinction between the kinds of general, aggregative decisions that are made at high levels of the organization, and the kinds of specific, item-by-item decisions that are made at low levels. We have already alluded to this distinction in the preceding example of a system for controlling inventory and production. When executives at high levels in such a system make decisions about "aggregate inventory," this mode of factoring the decision-making problem already involves radical simplification and approximation. For example, there is no single, well-defined total cost associated with a given total value of aggregate inventories. There will generally be different costs associated with each of the different kinds of items that make up the inventory (for example, different items may have different spoilage rates or obsolescence rates), and different probabilities and costs associated with stock-outs of each kind of item. Thus, a given aggregate inventory will have different costs depending on its composition in terms of individual items.

To design a system for making decisions about the aggregate work force, production rate, and inventories requires an assumption that the

---

[8] For some empirical evidence, see D. C. Dearborn and H. A. Simon, Selective Perception: A Note on the Departmental Identification of Executives, *Sociometry*, 21 (1958), 140–144.

aggregate inventory will never depart very far from a typical composition in terms of individual item types. The assumption is likely to be tolerable because subsidiary decisions are continually being made at other points in the organization about the inventories of individual items. These subsidiary decisions prevent an aggregate inventory from becoming severely unbalanced, hence make averages meaningful for the aggregate.

The assumption required for aggregation is not unlike that made by an engineer when he controls the temperature of a tank of water, with a single thermometer as indicator, knowing that sufficient mixing of the liquid in the tank is going on to maintain a stable pattern of temperature relations among its parts. With such a stable pattern it would be infeasible to control the process by means of a measurement of the average temperature.

If one set of decisions is made, on this approximate basis, about aggregate work force, production rate, and inventories, then these decisions can be used as constraints in making detailed decisions at subsidiary levels about the inventory or production of particular items. If the aggregate decision has been reached to make one million gallons of paint next month, then other decisions can be reached as to how much paint of each kind to make, subject to the constraint that the production quotas for the individual items should, when added together, total one million gallons.[9]

This simple example serves to elucidate how the whole mass of decisions that are continually being made in a complex organization can be viewed as an organized system. They constitute a system in which (1) particular decision-making processes are aimed at finding courses of action that are feasible or satisfactory in the light of multiple goals and constraints, and (2) decisions reached in any one part of the organization enter as goals or constraints into the decisions being made in other parts of the organization.

There is no guarantee that the decisions reached will be optimal with respect to any over-all organizational goal. The system is a loosely coupled one. Nevertheless, the results of the over-all system can be measured against one or more organizational goals, and changes can be made in the decision-making structure when these results are adjudged unsatisfactory.

Further, if we look at the decision-making structure in an actual organization, we see that it is usually put together in such a way as to insure that the decisions made by specialized units will be made in cognizance of the more general goals. Individual units are linked to the total

---

[9] A system of this kind is developed in detail in "Determining Production Quantities under Aggregate Constraints," in C. Holt, F. Modigliani, J. Muth, and H. A. Simon, *Planning Production, Inventories, and Work Force* (Englewood Cliffs, N.J., 1960).

system by production schedules, systems of rewards and penalties based on cost and profit goals, inventory limits, and so on. The loose coupling among the parts has the positive consequence of permitting specific constraints in great variety to be imposed on subsystems without rendering their decision-making mechanisms inoperative.

THE DECISION-MAKING SYSTEM AND ORGANIZATIONAL BEHAVIOR

In the previous sections great pains were taken to distinguish the goals and constraints (inducements and contributions) that motivate people to accept organizational roles from the goals and constraints that enter into their decision making when they are enacting those organizational roles. On the one hand, the system of personal inducements and contributions imposes constraints that the organization must satisfy if it is to survive. On the other hand, the constraints incorporated in the organizational roles, hence in what I have called the organizational decision-making system, are the constraints that a course of action must satisfy in order for the organization to adopt it.

There is no necessary *logical* connection between these two sets of constraints. After all, organizations sometimes fail to survive, and their demise can often be attributed to failure to incorporate all the important motivational concerns of participants among the constraints in the organizational decision-making system. For example, a major cause of small business failure is working capital shortage, a result of failure to constrain actions to those that are consistent with creditors' demands for prompt payment. Similarly, new products often fail because incorrect assumptions about the inducements important to consumers are reflected in the constraints that guide product design. (It is widely believed that the troubles of the Chrysler Corporation stemmed from the design premise that car purchasers were primarily interested in buying a good piece of machinery.)

In general, however, there is a strong empirical connection between the two sets of constraints, for the organizations we will usually observe in the real world—those that have succeeded in surviving for some time—will be precisely those which have developed organizational decision-making systems whose constraints guarantee that their actions maintain a favorable balance of inducements to contributions for their participants. The argument, an evolutionary one, is the same one we can apply to biological organisms. There is no logical requirement that the temperatures, oxygen concentrations, and so on, maintained in the tissues of a bird by its physiological processes should lie within the ranges required for its survival. It is simply that we will not often have opportunities for observing birds whose physiological regulators do not reflect these external constraints. Such birds are soon extinct.[10]

Thus, what the sociologist calls the functional requisites for survival can usually give us good clues for predicting organizational goals; however, if the functional requisites resemble the goals, the similarity is empirical, not definitional. What the goals are must be inferred from observation of the organization's decision-making processes, whether these processes be directed toward survival or suicide.

CONCLUSIONS

We can now summarize our answers to the question that introduced this paper: What is the meaning of the phrase "organizational goal"? First, we discovered that it is doubtful whether decisions are generally directed toward achieving a goal. It is easier, and clearer, to view decisions as being concerned with discovering courses of action that satisfy a whole set of constraints. It is this set, and not any one of its members, that is most accurately viewed as the goal of the action.

If we select any of the constraints for special attention, it is (a) because of its relation to the motivations of the decision maker, or (b) because of its relation to the search process that is generating or designing particular courses of action. Those constraints that motivate the decision maker and those that guide his search for actions are sometimes regarded as more "goal-like" than those that limit the actions he may consider or those that are used to test whether a potential course of action he has designed is satisfactory. Whether we treat all the constraints symmetrically or refer to some asymmetrically as goals is largely a matter of linguistic or analytic convenience.

When we come to organizational decisions, we observe that many, if not most, of the constraints that define a satisfactory course of action are associated with an organizational role and hence only indirectly with the personal motives of the individual who assumes that role. In this situation it is convenient to use the phrase organization goal to refer to constraints, or sets of constraints, imposed by the organizational role, which has only this indirect relation to the motives of the decision makers.

If we examine the constraint set of an organizational decision-making

---

[10] The relation between the functional requisites for survival and the actual constraints of the operating system is a central concept in W. R. Ashby's notion of a multistable system. See his *Design for a Brain* (2d ed.; New York, 1960).

system, we will generally find that it contains constraints that reflect virtually all the inducements and contributions important to various classes of participants. These constraints tend to remove from consideration possible courses of action that are inimical to survival. They do not, of course, by themselves, often fully determine the course of action.

In view of the hierarchical structure that is typical of most formal organizations, it is a reasonable use of language to employ organizational goal to refer particularly to the constraint sets and criteria of search that define roles at the upper levels. Thus it is reasonable to speak of conservation of forest resources as a principal goal of the U.S. Forest Service, or reducing fire losses as a principal goal of a city fire department. For high-level executives in these organizations will seek out and support actions that advance these goals, and subordinate employees will do the same or will at least tailor their choices to constraints established by the higher echelons with this end in view.

Finally, since there are large elements of decentralization in the decision making in any large organization, different constraints may define the decision problems of different positions or specialized units. For example, "profit" may not enter directly into the decision making of most members of a business organization. Again, this does not mean that it is improper or meaningless to regard profit as a principal goal of the business. It simply means that the decision-making mechanism is a loosely coupled system in which the profit constraint is only one among a number of constraints and enters into most subsystems only in indirect ways. It would be both legitimate and realistic to describe most business firms as directed toward profit making—subject to a number of side constraints—operating through a network of decision-making processes that introduces many gross approximations into the search for profitable courses of action. Further, the goal ascription does not imply that any employee is motivated by the firm's profit goal, although some may be.

This view of the nature of organization goals leaves us with a picture of organizational decision making that is not simple. But it provides us with an entirely operational way of showing, by describing the structure of the organizational decision-making mechanism, how and to what extent overall goals, like "profit" or "conserving forest resources" help to determine the actual courses of action that are chosen.

Subject Index

Aged
    psychological behavior of, 120
Aging
    psychology of, 125
Alternative generation 288
Alternative testing, 288
American Hospital Association, 3, 42
American Medical Association, 41
Arranging data, 262
Automatic choices, 265
Bayesian strategy, 241
Behavioral Sciences, 43
Blue Cross, 38
Bounded Rationality, 231
British Health System, 33
Budget projection, 195
Capitalism, 56
Capitalist production system, 55, 57
Casualties of medical progress, 14
Checking for consistency, 263
Choice criteria, 264
Chunking, 247
Code Observance, 211
Cognitive strain, 232
    determinants of, 232
    in information aggregation, 246
    in preference aggregation, 248

    in problem diagnosis, 245
    in problem formation, 244
    psychological determinants of, 234
Collateral systems, 54, 57
COMSAT, 155
Comparative analysis, 120
Consumption function, 102
Control
    domination, 84
    elective, 66
    process of, 66
    purpose of, 66
    system model developed, 79
    techniques for future-directed, 68
Corollaries of rational choice, 265
Data processing and analysis, 263
Decisions and Decision-making
    definition, 223, 257
    deliberative nature of, 223
    model, 224-227
    process, 258
    theory, 224
Decomposable matrices, 244
Deterministic outcomes
    multiple objectives, 273
    single objective, 272
Diagnostic risks, 16

Author Index